CYTOKINES AND GROWTH FACTORS IN BLOOD TRANSFUSION

DEVELOPMENTS IN HEMATOLOGY AND IMMUNOLOGY

Volume 32

The titles published in this series are listed at the end of this volume.

Cytokines and Growth Factors in Blood Transfusion

Proceedings of the Twentyfirst International Symposium on Blood Transfusion, Groningen 1996, organized by the Red Cross Blood Bank Noord Nederland

edited by

C. Th. SMIT SIBINGA and P. C. DAS

Red Cross Blood Bank Noord Nederland, The Netherlands

and

B. LÖWENBERG

Erasmus University,
Rotterdam, The Netherlands

KLUWER ACADEMIC PUBLISHERS
DORDRECHT / BOSTON / LONDON

A C.I.P. Catalogue record for this book is available from the Library of Congress.

ISBN 0-7923-4787-0

Published by Kluwer Academic Publishers,
P.O. Box 17, 3300 AA Dordrecht, The Netherlands.

Sold and distributed in the U.S.A. and Canada
by Kluwer Academic Publishers,
101 Philip Drive, Norwell, MA 02061, U.S.A.

In all other countries, sold and distributed
by Kluwer Academic Publishers Group,
P.O. Box 322, 3300 AH Dordrecht, The Netherlands.

Printed on acid-free paper

Printed in the Netherlands

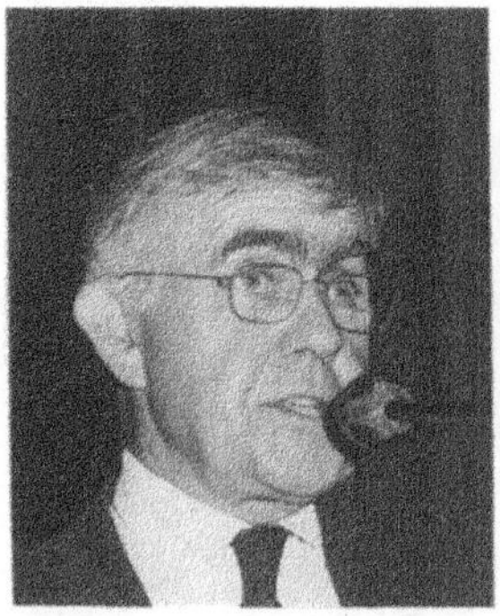

Dr. Cees Th. Smit Sibinga
Initiator and Organiser

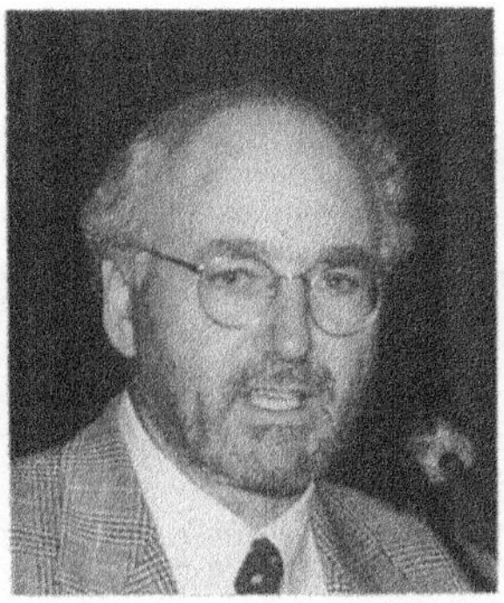

Prof. Dr. Bob Löwenberg
Chairman

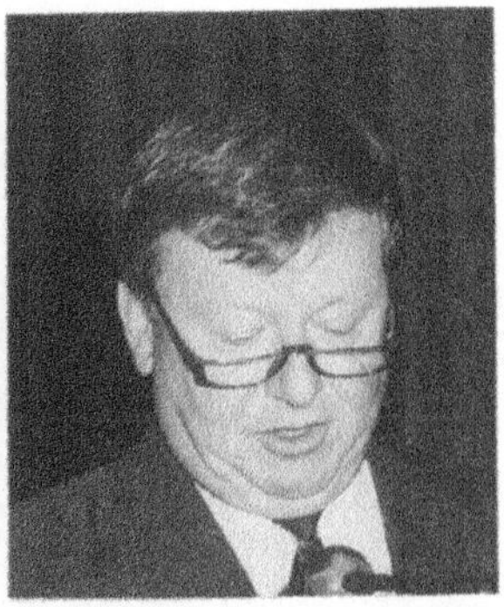

Mr. Hans Ouwerkerk
Mayor of Groningen,
opening address

Baxter

Acknowledgement

This publication has been made possible through the support of Baxter, which is gratefully acknowledged.

CONTENTS

IV. Future Potential of Cytokines and Growth Factors in Transfusion Medicine

MODERATORS AND SPEAKERS

Moderators

B. Löwenberg (chairman)	–	Daniël den Hoed Clinic, Rotterdam, NL
P.C. Das	–	Red Cross Blood Bank Noord Nederland, Groningen, NL
N.M. Heddle	–	McMaster University, Hamilton, Ontario, C
C.Th. Smit Sibinga	–	Red Cross Blood Bank Noord Nederland, Groningen, NL
H.J.C. de Wit	–	Red Cross Blood Bank Noord Nederland, Groningen, NL
J.Th.M. de Wolf	–	Academic Hospital Groningen, Department of Haematology, Groningen, NL

Speakers

T.A. Bock	–	University of Tübingen, Department of Haematology and Oncology, Tübingen, D
D.C. Dale	–	University of Washington, Seattle, WA, USA
H.M. Dupuis	–	University of Leiden, Department of Metamedica, Leiden, NL
M. Fujihara	–	Hokkaido Red Cross Blood Centre, Sapporo, J
L.T. Goodnough	–	Washington University School of Medicine, St. Louis, MO, USA
K. Kaushansky	–	University of Washington, Seattle, WA, USA
R. Mertelsmann	–	Albert-Ludwigs-Universität, Freiburg, D
N.H. Mulder	–	Academic Hospital Groningen, Department of Clinical Oncology, Groningen, NL

L. Muylle	– Blood Transfusion Centre Antwerp, Edegem, B
D.R. Rill	– St. Jude Children's Hospital, Division of BMT, Memphis, T, USA
J.W. Semple	– St. Michael's Hospital, Toronto, Ontario, C
P. Dreger	– Christian-Albrechts-Universität zu Kiel, Kiel, D
H. Spits	– Netherlands Cancer Institute, Amsterdam, NL
R.E.M. Toes	– University Hospital Leiden, Department of Immunohaematology, Leiden, NL
I.P. Touw	– Erasmus University Rotterdam, Department of Haematology, Rotterdam, NL
E. Vellenga	– Academic Hospital Groningen, Department of Haematology, Groningen, NL

OPENING ADDRESS

Ladies and gentlemen,

It is a great honour for me as mayor of the city of Groningen to welcome you here. Your visit is part of a commendable tradition on which people with scientific and professional ambitions have been meeting one another here for more than two decades. As a city with ambitions, because that is what we are, we see ourselves in you. The work of the Red Cross Blood Bank in the northern Netherlands under the supervision of its medical director Dr. Cees Smit Sibinga is making a significant contribution to these ambitions. It is putting Groningen on the map as a result of which the northern part of the Netherlands is not only receiving national recognition, but also the recognition it deserves elsewhere in the world, internationally. As one of the large urban centres in the nothern Netherlands we are especially glad to make room for know-how and quality. This, in addition to culture and environment, are two of our trade marks. We have invested a great deal in our city's beauty and quality of life, but just as you we also know that quality is not something that one attains at anyone point in time. It is actually something that demands ongoing maintenance and the making of adjustments to new challenges. Among other things it is this glimpse into the future that makes your annual gatherings here in Groningen so worthwhile and makes them an example of what the dedication, required to obtain knowledge and know-how, can provide to an activity which is difficult to control. When I call this dedication an important gain from this symposium, I do not do so by chance. In these times too often I feel the lack of a contribution which could be made by scientists and professionals to help solve the problems which cities in the world are increasingly having to face. Naturally, there are signs that the problems of society including health care are being taken seriously. Here and there important contributions are already being made. I am making a plea, here in the midst of so many influential scientists and professionals, for an improvement in the matching together the agendas of city politics and the relevant institutions for research and development. The degree to which we succeed in doing something about the problems of today's city as the place, where the gaps in our society make themselves apparent, will be a determining factor in the degree of which we can get to continue to appeal sucessfully for solidarity. Indifference, apathy and aloofness all form the crux of the symptom to which society must call a halt or be rupt fundamentally of its own strength.

Ladies and gentlemen, do not assume from what I am saying however, that

I would allow myself to be persuaded by pessimism. I continue to have great confidence in the power of solidarity and in the degree to which we can still appeal to that solidarity. It is for good reason that the donor pool of our blood bank has doubled since 1976 to its present 80,000 registered volunteer blood donors coming from every stratum of the population. To take care of the needs of 1.7 million inhabitants, this is a good percentage, but we can always use more.

Ladies and gentlemen, I know that the field of knowledge involving blood banks is continually on the move. Quality, safety and efficiency are key words, that not only involve the scientific and professional value of the work, but also effect its organisation, design and management. Such changes occur in a tempo which for one person might be too fast, but for another could be too slow, but a change is inevitable. I am confident that your scientific and professional curiosity will bring you solutions. Therefore I wish you success with your 21st international symposium on blood transfusion. May it meet with your high expectations. Welcome in our city of Groningen. Thank you.

Hans Ouwerkerk,
mayor of Groningen

I. FUNDAMENTAL ASPECTS OF CYTOKINES AND GROWTH FACTORS

THE ROLE OF THE COMMON GAMMA CHAIN OF THE IL-2, IL-4, IL-7 AND IL-15 RECEPTORS IN DEVELOPMENT OF LYMPHOCYTES. CONSTITUTIVE EXPRESSION OF Bcl-2 DOES NOT RESCUE THE DEVELOPMENTAL DEFECTS IN GAMMA COMMON-DEFICIENT MICE

B. Blom[1], H. Spits[1], P. Krimpenfort[2]

Introduction

It is firmly established that cytokines are involved in development of hematopoietic cells. Until recently it was not known whether cytokines are involved in development of lymphoid cells. Initially, interleukin (IL)-2 and IL-4 were considered to be candidates essential for lymphoid development. However, this turned out not to be the case since mice deficient for IL-2 [1], IL-4 [2] or both [3] had no obvious defects with regard to development of T and B cells. Nonetheless, it became clear that cytokines do play an essential role in T cell development when the molecular defect underlying the X chromosome linked severe combined immunodeficiency (X-SCID) was determined [4]. These patients have no T or NK cells but B cells are present in normal numbers. It turned out that these patients have mutations in the gamma chain of the IL-2 receptor complex [4]. As it was already known that IL-2 is not essential for T cell development, it was suspected that this component of the IL-2R was also part of receptors for other cytokines. This suspicion was confirmed soon thereafter when it was found that the IL-2Rγ chain is also a component of the receptors of IL-4, IL-7, IL-9 and IL-15 [5-7]. Therefore, the IL-2Rγ chain is now commonly referred to as the gamma common (γc) chain. Studies with IL-7 [8] and IL-7Rα chain deficient mice [9] have made clear that IL-7 is the critical γc ligand involved in T cell development. Like the γc deficient mice [10], these mice have a thymus that is only 10% in size of the wild type thymus. TCRαβ+ T cells are present in the periphery but the number of these cells is strongly reduced. Almost no TCRγδ+ cells are found in the IL-7Rα –/– mice, indicating that IL-7 is more critical for development of these latter cells than for TCRαβ+ cells. The IL-7 and IL-7Rα deficient mice have also a strong block in development of B cells, but normal numbers of NK cells are present [8,9]. Gamma common null mice have the same defects in T and B cell development as IL-7 and IL-7Rα null mice but also lack NK cells [10,ll]. Which γc ligand is critical for development of NK cells has not yet been definitively determined. Plum et al. have

1. Department of Immunology of the Netherlands Cancer Institute. Plesmanlaan 121, 1066 CX Amsterdam, Netherlands.
2. Department of Genetics of the Netherlands Cancer Institute. Plesmanlaan 121, 1066 CX Amsterdam, Netherlands.

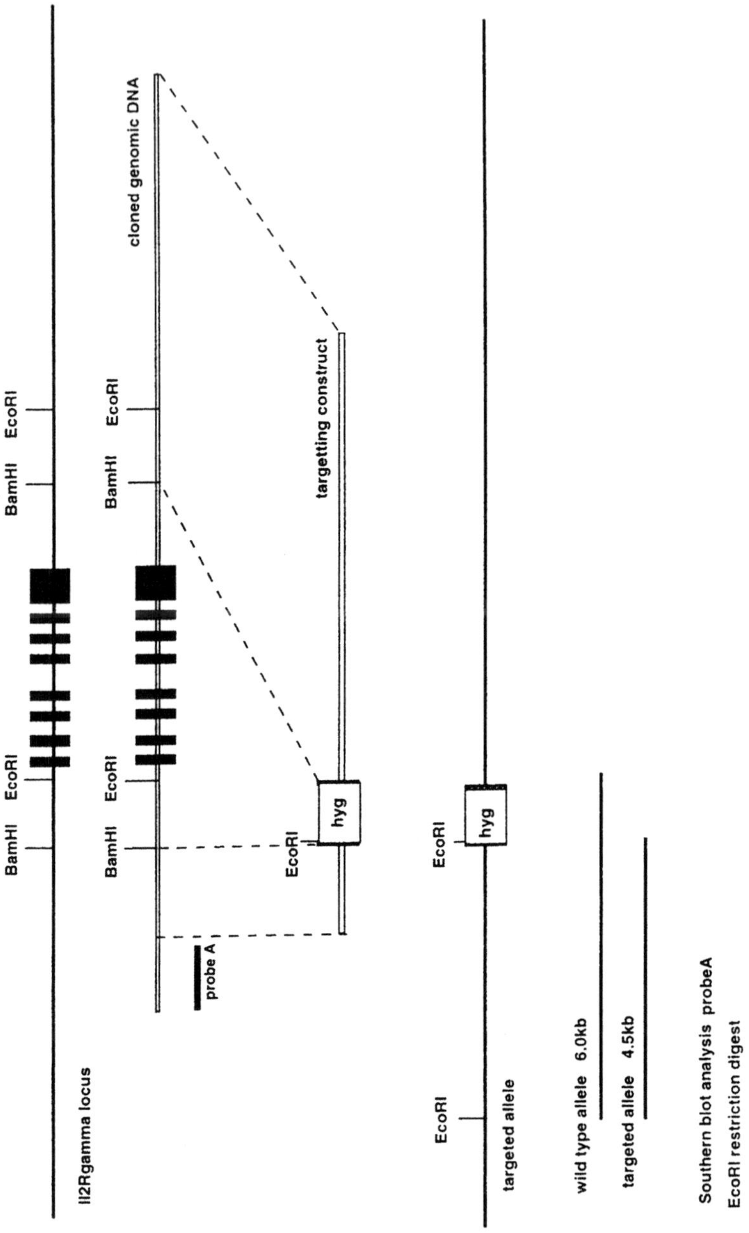

Figure 1. Inactivation of the gc gene by homologous recombination.

found that antibodies against IL-7 or the IL-7Rα chain inhibit development of human CD34+ fetal liver cells in a fetal thymic organ culture [12], indicating that IL-7 is critical for T cell development in humans as well. At what stages IL-7 affects T cell development in humans is, however, not known. In contrast to the requirement of IL-7 for B cell development in the mouse, IL-7 is not critical for development of B cells in humans [13].

A critical question is whether hematopoietic factors maintain the viability of cells in certain stages of development thereby allowing further development to proceed or whether the cytokines induce differentiation. A way to investigate this is to analyse the effect of cytokines on differentiation of progenitor cells overexpressing the Bcl-2 gene [14]. Bcl-2 can protect cells against apoptosis [15]. If the γc chain is important just for survival of T cell progenitor cells, we can expect that introduction of Bcl-2 restores the defect caused by the γc deficiency. If, alternatively, the γc chain is important for differentiation, we might expect that Bcl-2 has no effect on lymphoid development in the γc null mice. In this paper we have analysed Bcl-2 transgenic mice deficient for the γc chain.

Materials and methods

Generation of γc null mice

The targeting construct used to generate ES cells with the null mutation of the γc locus is depicted in Figure 1. ES cells were transfected and selected in hygromycin and cloned. Clones were analysed for the presence of homologous recombinations by Southern blotting. Chimeric 129 mice were generated following blastocyst injection of the targeted ES cells and implantation into pseudo pregnant foster mothers. Chimeric mice were back crossed to generate γc null male mice. Bcl-2 Tg gc null mice were generated by crossing Bcl-2 females [16, obtained from S. Korsmeyer] with γc null males. The mice were analysed at 2.5 weeks of age.

Flow cytometric analysis

Single cell suspensions were made of thymi, spleen and bone marrow cells. Erythrocytes, contaminating spleen cell suspensions were lysed by treatment with NH_4Cl. Before incubation with mAbs, the cells were incubated with 2% normal mouse serum to block Fc receptors. Cells were incubated for 30 min's with mAbs conjugated with fluorochromes (phycoerythrin or FITC) and washed twice before analysis on a FacScan (Becton Dickinson, San José, CA). Data were analysed with the Cell Quest program (Becton Dickinson). The NK cell-specific antibody DX5 was a kind gift of Dr. Lewis Lanier, DNAX Research Institute, Palo Alto, CA). All other antibodies were purchased from Pharmingen (San Diego, CA).

Cyotoxic activity of NK cells

Cytotoxic NK activity of spleen cells was measured with a standard ^{51}Cr release assay. Varied numbers of spleen cells were added to 2000 labelled YAC-1 target

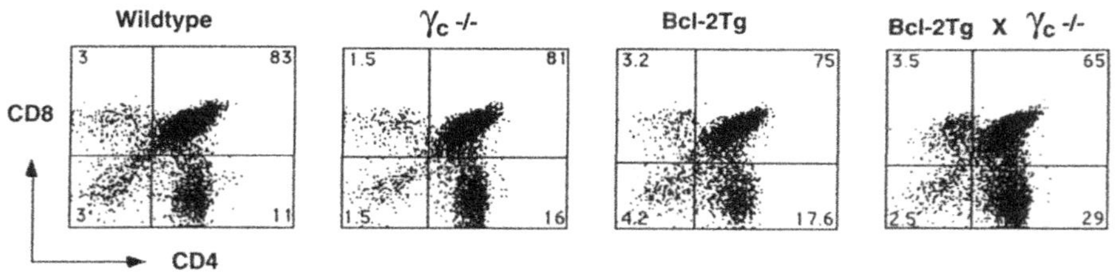

Figure 2. Expression of CD4 and CD8 of thymocytes of wildetype, γc null, Bcl-2 Tg and Tgx gc null littermates.

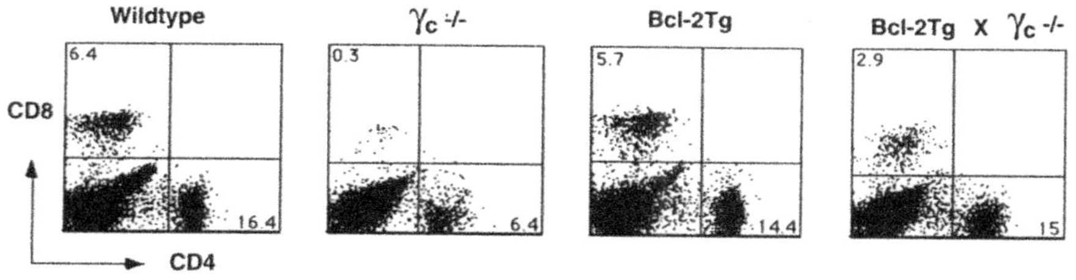

Figure 3. Expression of CD4 and CD8 on spleen cells of wildtype, γc null, Bcl-2 Tg and Bcl-2 Tgx gc null littermates.

cells in round bottomed wells of a 96 wells plate (Costar, Badhoevedorp, Netherlands) and the plates were incubated for 4 hr. Supernatants were harvested and measured with a scintillation counter. Percentage specific release was determined with the formula: release of the sample-spontaneous release/maximum release-spontaneous release. Maximum and spontaneous releases were determined by incubating the labelled cells in 1% Triton X 100 and medium respectively.

Results

Effect of constitutive expression of Bcl-2 on thymic development in γc deficient mice

Disruption of the γc chain results in defects in T, B and NK cell development. To investigate whether these defects are caused by disruption of the differentiation processes or by diminished survival of progenitor cells, γc deficient mice were crossed with Bcl-2 transgenic animals. We have analysed the mice at 2.5 weeks of age. The Bcl-2 Tg γc null mice were as healthy as their wild type, Bcl-2 TG, and γc null littermates. The number of thymocytes and the phenotype of the thymocytes of these animals were compared with those of wt and Bcl-2 Tg animals (Fig. 1). Thymic cellularity of the Bcl-2 Tg γc null mice (30×10^6) was increased slightly compared to the γc null littermate (20×10^6). Nonetheless the number of thymocytes of the γc null and the γc null/Bcl-2 Tg animals were still much lower respectively wild type and Bcl-2 Tg animals (350 and 376×10^6 cells per thymus respectively). Comparison of the proportions of CD4+, CD8+ single positive (SP), CD4+CD8+ double positive (DP) and of CD3+ cells in the thymi of these animals revealed that constitutive expression of Bcl-2 results in a slight increase of SP thymocytes at cost of the DP (Fig. 2). This latter effect is even more apparent in thymi of older mice (data not shown).

Constitutive expression of Bcl-2 results in increased survival of CD3+ CD8+ cells in the spleen of young (2.5 weeks old) mice

Although development of T cells in γc null mice is delayed and the cellularity of the thymus is reduced tenfold, these mice have T cells in the periphery. At 2.5 week of age, the numbers of splenic cells are approximately 10-15 fold lower than in wild type animals (11×10^6 vs 80×10^6) but when becoming older these mice accumulate T cells in the periphery and by the age of 7-9 months the number of T cells reaches wild type levels (results not shown). Despite that young γc null mice have T cells, the relative proportion of CD8+ T cells is 20 fold lower than in wild type animals, while that of CD4+ T cells is only 2.5 fold lower (Fig. 3). Figure 3 shows that constitutive expression of Bcl-2 in γc null mice significantly increases the relative proportion of CD8+ T cells (2.9%) compared to γc null mice without Bcl-2 (0.3%). The CD4:CD8 ratio in the γc null Bcl-2 Tg mice (5:1) was higher than in wild type animals (2.5:1) but much lower than in γc null mice (20:1). These data indicate that Bcl-2 expression results in better survival of CD4+ and CD8+ T cells in the spleen of γc null mice. This effect is more pronounced with CD8+ than with CD4+ T cells.

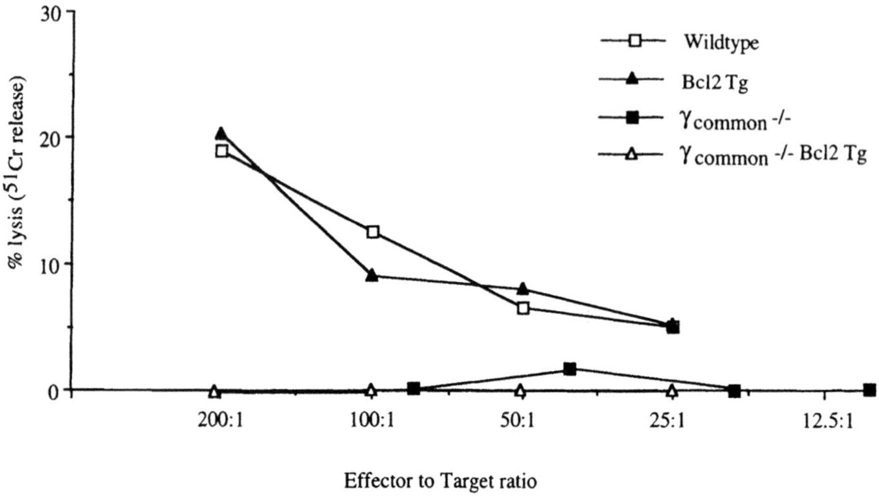

Figure 4. NK activities of spleen cells of γc null × Bcl-2 Tg mice and their wt, Bcl-2 Tg and γc null littermates. The percentages of DX5+NK cells in these spleen cell populations were: γc null × Bcl-2 Tg: <0.3%, γc null: <0.5%, wt: 2.9% and Bcl-2 Tg: 1.5%.

NK development is not restored by expression of Bcl-2 in γc null mice.

NK cells are absent in γc null mice. We could also not detect NK cells in the bone marrow and spleen of γc null × Bcl-2 Tg animals using the NK-specific antibody DX5. In contrast to the wt and the Bcl-2 Tg animals, no NK activity against the NK-sensitive target cell YAC- 1 could be detected (Fig. 4). These data indicate that Bcl-2 Tg is unable to rescue the development of NK cells and suggest that a γc ligand is essential for differentiation of NK cells.

Discussion

The present study addressed the question whether the disturbances of T and NK cell development, caused by deficiency of the γc chain of the IL-2, IL-4, IL-7, IL-9 and IL-15 receptors, are due to diminished survival of progenitor cells or by intrinsic differentiation defects. Our data show that Bcl-2 increases the cellularity of the thymus, but does not significantly alter the relative proportions of the SP and DP thymocytes indicating that the γc ligands involved in T cell development are promoting survival of thymic progenitor cells and their progeny. Since Bcl-2 does not restore cellularity of the thymus to wild type levels we conclude that the γc ligand, involved in development of T cells (presumably IL-7), is important for expansion of the progenitor cells and not just for survival of these cells. Gamma common deficiency results in defects in CD8+ T cells. DiSanto and collaborators have crossed the γ null mutant mice with mice expressing a transgenic T cell receptor specific for the male antigen HY [17]. They demonstrated that, although the CD8+ TCR Tg cells developed normally and are present in the thymus, they are not detectable in the spleen and other peripheral organs. This could be due to a defect in the ability to migrate out of the thymus or to a survival defect. We found that the number of CD8+ cells in the spleen of young mice is strongly diminished compared to that of CD4+ T cells. Bcl-2 expression results in a significant increase of CD8+ cells in the spleen of young γc null mice, indicating that a γc ligand is important for survival of CD8+ T cells in the periphery. It is presently not clear which ligand that Bcl-2 expression has no effect on development of B cells, but an accumulation of pro B cells was observed in some, but not in all, mice (results not shown). These observations indicate that a γc ligand is important for driving differentiation of B cells. It is most likely that IL-7 is this ligand. The notion that IL-7 is essential for differentiation of B cells and not just for survival of the B cell progenitors and their progeny, is supported by findings of Venkitaraman who demonstrated that IL-7 is implicated in induction of rearrangements of the Ig genes [18]. It is of note here that the γc chain is not critical for development of B cells in humans. Patients suffering an X linked SCID due to mutations in the γc gene, have normal or even elevated numbers of B cells [19]. Recent data have made clear that B cells can differentiate *in vitro* without IL-7 [13]. Identification of the cytokines important for development of human B cells will be one challenge for the future. The γc chain is essential for development of NK cells, since virtually no NK cells are found in γc null mice. Our data demonstrate that Bcl-2 fails to rescue NK developmental effect. This indicates that a γc ligand is essential for induction of NK cell development. The nature of the critical ligand is yet unknown. However, IL-2, IL-4 and IL-7 are not involved in development of NK cells, since mice deficient for these cytokines do have NK cells. Recently it was found that IL-2R beta null mice also lack NK cells [20]. IL-15 is probably the γc ligand essential for NK development, since not only IL-2 but also IL-15 binds to a γc/IL-2Rβ complex [21]. This notion is supported by the findings that IL-15 can drive NK cell development *in vitro* [22]. Definitive assessment of the role of IL-15 in NK cell development should await analysis of IL-15 deficient mice.

Acknowledgements

We thank Dr. A Berns for support, Dr. S Korsmeyer for providing the Bcl-2 Tg animals and Dr. L. L. Lanier for providing us with the DX5 antibody.

References

1. Schorle H, Holtschke T, Hunig T, Schimpl A, Horak I. Development and function of T cells in mice rendered interleukin-2 deficient by gene targeting. Nature 1991;352: 621-24.
2. Kuhn R, Rajewski K, Muller W. Generation and analysis of Interleukin-4 deficient mice. Science 1991;254:707-10.
3. Sadlack B, Kuhn R, Schorle H, Rajewski K, Muller W, Horak I. Development and proliferation of lymphocytes in mice deficient for both interleukins-2 and -4. Eur J Immunol 1994;24:281-84.
4. Noguchi M, Yi H, Rosenblatt HM, et al. Interleukin-2 receptor gamma chain mutation results in X-linked severe combined immunodeficiency in humans. Cell 1993;73: 147-57.
5. Noguchi M, Nakamura Y, Russell SM, et al. Interleukin-2 receptor gamma chain: A functional component of the interleukin-7 receptor. Science 1993;262: 1877-80.
6. Kondo M, Takeshita T, Ishii N, et al. Sharing of the interleukin-2 (IL-2) receptor gamma chain between receptors for IL-2 and IL-4. Science 1993;262: 1874-77.
7. Russell SM, Keegan AD, Harada N, et al. Interleukin-2 receptor γ chain: A functional component of the interleukin-4 receptor. Science 1993;262:1880-83.
8. Von Freeden B, Jeffry U, Vieira P, et al. Lymphopenia in interleukin (IL)-7 gene-deleted mice identifies IL-7 as a nonredundant cytokine. J Exp Med 1995;181:1519-26.
9. Peschon JJ, Morrissey PJ, Grahstein KH, et al. Early lymphocyte expansion is severely impaired in interleukin 7 receptor-deficient mice. J Exp Med 1994;1804:1955-60.
10. DiSanto JP, Muller W, Guy GD, Fischer A, Rajewsky K. Lymphoid development in mice with a targeted deletion of the interleukin 2 receptor gamma chain. Proc Natl Acad Sci USA 1995;92:377-81.
11. Cao X, Shores EW, Hu LJ, et al. Defective lymphoid development in mice lacking expression of the common cytokine receptor gamma chain. Immunity 1995;2:223-38.
12. Plum J, De Smedt M, Leclercq G, Verhasselt B, Vanderkerckhove B. Interleukin-7 is a critical growth factor in early human T-cell development. Blood 1996;88:4239-45.
13. Prieyl JA, LeBien TW. Interleukin 7 independent development of human B cells. Proc Natl Acad Sci USA 1996;93:10348-53.
14. Fairbairn LJ, Cowling GJ, Reipert BM, Dexter TM. Suppression of apoptosis allows differentiation and development of a multipotent hemopoietic cell line in the absence of added growth factors. Cell 1993;74:823-32.
15. Yang E, Korsmeyer SJ. Molecular thanatopsis: A discourse on the Bcl-2 family and cell death. Blood 1996;88:386-401.
16. McDonnell TJ, Nunez G, Platt FM, et al. Deregulated Bcl-2-immunoglobulin transgene expands a resting but responsive immunoglohulin M and D-expressing B-cell population. Mol Cell Biol 1990;10:1901-7.
17. DiSanto JP, Guy GD, Fisher A, Tarakhovsky A. Critical role for the common cytokine receptor gamma chain in intrathymic and peripheral T cell selection. J Exp Med 1996; 183:1111-18.
18. Corcoran AE, Smart FM, Cowling RJ, Crompton T, Owen MJ, Venkitaraman AR. The interleukin-7 receptor alpha chain transmits distinct signals for proliferation and differ-

entiation during B lymphopoiesis. EMBO J 1996;15:1924-32.

19. Voss SD, Hong R, Sondel PM. Severe combined immunodeficiency, interleukin-2 (IL-2), and the IL-2 receptor: experiments of nature continue to point the way. Blood 1994;83:626-35.
20. Suzuki H, Duncan GS, Takimoto H, Mak TW. Abnormal development of intestinal intraepithelial lymphocytes and peripheral natural killer cells in mice lacking the IL-2 receptor beta chain. J Exp Med 1997;185:499-505.
21. Grabstein KH, Eisenman J, Shanebeck K, et al. Cloning of a T cell growth factor that interacts with the β chain of the Interleukin-2 receptor. Science 1994;264:965-68.
22. Puzanov IJ, Bennett M, Kumar V. IL-15 can substitute for the marrow micro-environment in the differentiation of natural killer cells. J Immunol 1996;157:4282-85.

MOLECULAR MECHANISMS INVOLVED IN THE CONTROL OF DIFFERENTIAL CYTOKINE EXPRESSION IN HUMAN MONOCYTES

L.M.L. Tuyt[1], W.H.A. Dokter[2], E. Vellenga[1]

During the last few years a tremendous increase has been obtained in our knowledge of cytokines. Apart from the identification of new cytokines we have reached a better understanding of cytokine gene regulation as well as of signal transduction pathways leading to cytokine gene expression. One of the intriguing phenomena of the regulation of cytokines is the specificity in effects of stimulatory agents which has been observed in different haematopoietic cells. This differential regulation of cytokines is most extensively studied in human monocytes.

The main cytokines produced by monocytes are interleukin-1 (IL-1), IL-6, Tumour Necrosis Factor (TNF), Granulocyte-Colony Stimulating Factor (G-CSF), Macrophage-CSF (M-CSF), and GM-CSF [1]. Illustrative for the differential regulation of cytokines in monocytes is the observation that different signals are required for the production of G-CSF, M-CSF, and IL-6 [2,3]. IL-3, GM-CSF, and interferon-γ (IFN-γ) have been shown to selectively induce M-CSF mRNA expression, whereas G-CSF and IL-6 transcripts were observed in response to IL-1 or lipopolysaccharide (LPS) stimulation [3,9]. The calcium ionophore A23187 appeared to induce both M-CSF and IL-6 mRNA expression in the human monocytic cell line Mono Mac 6, indicating that M-CSF and IL-6 are both expressed in response to intracellular Ca^{2+} mobilization. It was furthermore observed that costimulation of the protein kinase C (PKC) or PKA dependent pathways (with phorbol myristate acetate (PMA) and dibutyryl cAMP (DBcAMP) respectively) had contrasting effects on M-CSF and IL-6 gene expression. Costimulation of these cells with A23187 plus the phorbolester PMA resulted in a upregulation of M-CSF mRNA whereas the IL-6 mRNA was down-regulated. Conversely, costimulation with A23187 plus DBcAMP resulted in a down-regulation of M-CSF mRNA and an upregulation of IL-6 mRNA.

1. Division of Haematology, Department of Medicine, University of Groningen, The Netherlands.
2. Center for Biomedical Technology, Department of Medicine, University of Groningen, The Netherlands.

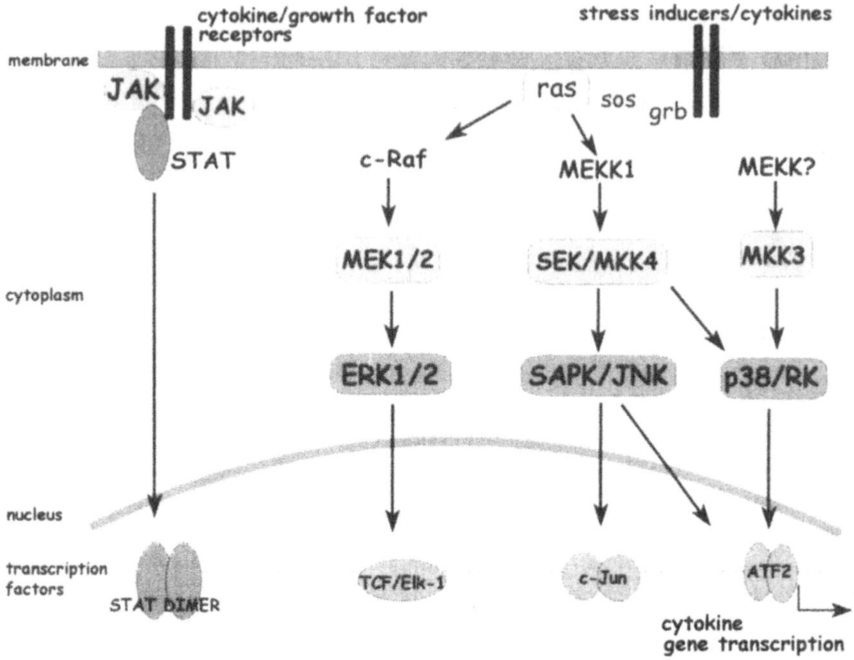

Figure 1. Schematic representation of four signaling cascades important in the regulation of cytokine gene expression. In the JAK/STAT pathway the interaction of a cytokine or growth factor to its cognate receptor is followed by the oligomerization of the receptor chains. The activation of the JAK proteins results in the phosphorylation of specific tyrosine residues within the intracellular part of the cytokine receptor which then serve as docking sites for STAT proteins. The subsequent phosphorylation of the receptor-associated STAT proteins by JAK results in dissociation of the STAT proteins from the receptor, dimerization of the STAT molecules and translocation into the nucleus where the dimers will bind to their recognition sequences on the promoters of the responsive genes. Each of the three MAPK pathways consists of a cascade of protein kinases ultimately resulting in the phosphorylation and activation of transcription factors and subsequent activation of gene transcription. The MAPK pathways described so far are the ERK1/ERK2 cascade, the JNK/SAPK and the p38pathway.

The specificity of cytokine production is not only demonstrated by the differ--ential effects of the stimuli applied, but is also underscored by a phenomenon which is termed "priming". G-CSF mRNA expression and secretion by monocytic cells is triggered by LPS and by IL-1 [3]. Stimulation of monocytes with IFN-γ did not result in the expression of G-CSF mRNA expression. However, when monocytes were pretreated with IFN-γ for a short period of time followed by LPS stimulation, the stimulatory effects of LPS on mRNA and protein level were potentiated by IFN-γ. Similar phenomena were observed regarding IL-6 mRNA expression in monocytic cells [10]. IL-3 alone was not capable of inducing the expression of IL-6 mRNA in contrast to the IL-1 mRNA expression. However, monocytes primed with IL-3 and followed by LPS stimulation demonstrated a significant increase in the IL-6 mRNA expression and secretion compared to stimulation with LPS alone. The induction of cytokine mRNA expression is dependent on two regulatory mechanisms, namely the transcription rate of the particular gene and the post-transcriptional stabilization of the mRNA [11]. For G-CSF, for instance, it was demonstrated that both the transcription rate of the G-CSF gene and the half-life of the G-CSF mRNA were increased after stimulation with IFN-γ and LPS compared to LPS treatment alone.

Induction of the transcription rate of a certain gene is indicative of changes in the expression of transcription factors involved in the regulation of the gene. For IL-6, among others, much information has become available about the transcription factors which are involved in the activation of the IL-6 promoter and thus in the IL-6 gene regulation [12,13,14]. Three transcription factors which are important in the IL-6 promoter activity are Activator Protein-1 (AP-1), Nuclear Factor kappa B (NF-κB), and NF-IL6 [15-20]. AP-1 consists of heterodimers of proteins of the jun and of the fos family [21]. The best known heterodimer is the combination of c-jun and c-fos. In several reports it has been implicated as a negative regulator of the IL-6 promoter activity [22]. NF-κB has been shown to be a transcription factor for many cytokine genes, including IL-1, IL-6, M-CSF, and G-CSF [23-27]. It consists of a homo- or heterodimer of the Rel protein family and is constitutively present in the cytosol of cells. A heterodimer between p65 and p105 is the most common and best described form of NF-κB. In the cytosol it is bound to the inhibitor protein IκB. After activation of the cell IκB is phosphorylated and degraded, p105 is processed and an active p65/p50 heterodimer is translocated to the nucleus to bind to the κB-sites of the appropriate promoters. NF-IL6 is a nuclear factor belonging to the CCAAT/enhancer binding protein (C/EBP) family whose mRNA synthesis is regulated by IL-6 and by other cytokines [18,19].

The underlying mechanism of differential cytokine regulation by different stimuli most likely involves the activation of a different set of transcription factors. With regard to the difference between LPS and IL-3 in mediating IL-6 mRNA expression it was demonstrated that IL-3 induced the p50 subunit of NF-κB, whereas LPS induced a heterodimer of p50 and p65 [10]. Homodimers of p50 will bind to the appropriate κB-site but will not elicite transactivation of the IL-6 promoter, whereas the p50/p65 heterodimer is supposed to be the active form of NF-κB. No difference was found regarding the induction of AP-1 and NF-IL6, suggesting that NF-κB is indeed a key factor in mediating IL-6 mRNA expression.

Activation of transcription factors is preceded by a sequence of protein phosphorylation, termed "signal transduction". Binding of a ligand, for example a cytokine, to its cognate receptor initiates a cascade of events ultimately resulting in gene transcription. A few of the classical signal transduction pathways are intracellular Ca^{2+}, Protein Kinase C (PKC), PKA, and Arachidonic Acid metabolism. More recently, a number of additional second messenger pathways have been characterized which appear involved in the regulation of cytokine expression. In the JAK/STAT pathway ligand binding and receptor dimerization leads to the tyrosine phosphorylation of associated cytoplasmic protein tyrosine kinases belonging to the JAK (Janus kinase) family [28-30]. Four family members have been identified in mammalians, namely JAK1, JAK2, JAK3, and TYR2. JAKs phosphorylate and activate the STAT (Signal Transducer and Activator of Transcription) proteins, which subsequently dimerize and translocate to the nucleus. Homo- or heterodimers of STAT proteins bind to specific DNA sequences in promoter regions of responsive genes and stimulate transcription. Seven members of the STAT family have been identified until now (STAT1-STAT6, and LIL-STAT). G-CSF, IL-6, and IL-10 for example, activate STAT3 [31,32]; IL-6, IL-1, and LPS induce LIL-STAT phosphorylation, whereas IFN-γ affects STAT1 activation [33-35]. IL-4 has been demonstrated to be the sole activator of STAT6 [36].

A second recently characterized group of signaling pathways involved in cytokine-induced signal transduction and regulation of cytokine gene expression are the mitogen-activated protein kinase (MAPK) pathways. Three MAPK pathways have been described in mammalian cells and they consist of a cascade of protein kinases which lead to phosphorylation and activation of transcription factors and subsequently to activation of gene expression [37,38]. The most extensively characterized of the mammalian MAP kinases is the RAF-MEK-ERK (extracellular-regulated kinase) cascade [39,40]. ERK1 and ERK2 (the 44 kDa and 42 kDa isoforms respectively) can be activated when cells are exposed, among others, to growth factors and phorbol esters. The second MAPK pathway comprises the stress-activated protein kinases (SAPK), which are activated by cellular stresses such as heat shock, sodium arsenite, UV radiation and osmotic shock, but also by bacterial endotoxins and pro-inflammatory cyokines [41-43]. The SAP kinases are only poorly activated in response to growth factors. The third distinct kinase, known as reactivating kinase (RK) or p38, is also stimulated in response to stress, bacterial endotoxin and pro-inflammatory cytokines. Both SAPK and p38 are kinases in the onset of apoptosis.

Although the precise role of the various signal transduction pathways in the regulation of the individual cytokines has not yet been completely resolved, it is clear that the different intracellular signaling pathways control the activation of the different subsets of transcription factors which in turn results in differential expression of cytokines in monocytic cells: this event will subsequently give the cell the opportunity to respond in many ways on external activation signals.

REFERENCES

1. Nathan CF. Secretory products of macrophages. J Clin Invest 1987;79:319-26.
2. De Wit H, Esselink MT, Halie MR, Vellenga E. Differential regulation of M-CSF and IL-6 gene expression in monocytic cells. Br J Haematol 1994;86:259-64.
3. De Wit H, Dokter WHA, Esselink MT, Halie MR, Vellenga E. Interferon-γ enhances the LPS-induced G-CSF gene expression in human adherent monocytes which is regulated at transcriptional and post-transcriptional level. Exp Haematol 1993;21:785-90.

4. Horiguchi J, Warren MK, Kufe D. Expression of macrophage specific colony-stimulating factor in human monocytes treated with granulocyte-macrophage colony-stimulating factor. Blood 1987;69:1259-61.
5. Vellenga E, Rambaldi A, Ernst TJ, Ostapovicz D, Griffin JD. Independent regulation of M-CSF and G-CSF gene expression in human monocytes. Blood 1988; 71:1529-32.
6. Rambaldi A, Young DC, Griffin JD. Expression of the M-CSF (CSF-1) gene by human monocytes. Blood 1987;69:1409-13.
7. Oster W, Lindemann A, Horn S, Mertelsmann R, Herrmann F. Tumour necrosis factor (TNF)-alpha but not TNF-beta induces secretion of colony-stimulating factor for macrophages (CSF-1) by human monocytes. Blood 1987;70:1700-3.
8. Bauer J, Ganter U, Geiger T, et al. Regulation of interleukin-6 expression in cultured human blood monocytes and monocyte derived macrophages. Blood 1988; 72:1134-40.
9. Tosato G, Jones KD. Interleukin-1 induces interleukin-6 production in peripheral blood monocytes. Blood 1990;75:1305-10.
10. Tuyt LML, de Wit H, Koopmans SB, Sierdsema SJ, Vellenga E. Effects of IL-3 and LPS on transcription factors involved in the regulation of IL-6 mRNA. Br J Haematol 1996; 92:521-29.
11. Bernstein P, Ross J. Poly(A) binding protein and the regulation of mRNA stability. Trends biochem sci 1989;14:373-77.
12. Rambaldi A, Bettoni S, Rossi V, et al. Transcriptional and post-transcriptional regulation of IL-1ß, IL-6 and TNF-α genes in chronic lymphocytic leukaemia. Br J Haematol 1993;83:204-11.
13. Pleszczynski MR, Stankova J. Leukotriene B4 enhances interleukin-6 (IL-6) production and IL-6 messenger RNA acuumulation in human monocytes in vitro: transcriptional and post-transcriptional mechanisms. Blood 1992;80:1004-11.
14. Sehgal PB. Regulation of IL-6 gene expression. Res immunol 1992;143:724-34.
15. Tanabe O, Akira S, Kamiya T, et al. Genomic structure of the murine IL-6 gene: high degree conservation of potential regulatory sequences between mouse and human. J Immunol 1988;141:3875-81.
16. Shimizu H, Mitomo K, Watanabe T, Okamoto S, Yamamoto K. Involvement of a NF-κB-like transcription factor in the activation of ithe interleukin-6 gene by inflammatory lymphokines. Mol Cell Biol 1990;10:561-68.
17. Libermann TA, Baltimore D. Activation of interleukin-6 gene expression through the NF-κB transcription factor. Mol Cell Biol 1990;10:2327-34.
18. Akira S, Isshiki H, Nakajima T, et al. Regulation of expression of the interleukin-6 gene: structure and function of the transcription factor NF-IL6. CIBA Found Symp 1992;167:47-67.
19. Akira S, Isshiki H, Sugita T, et al. A nuclear factor for IL-6 expression (NF-IL6) is a member of a C/EBP family. EMBO J 1990;9:1897-906.
20. Isshiki H, Akira S, Tanabe O, et al. Constitutive and IL-1-inducible factors interact with the IL-1-response element in the IL-6 gene. Mol Cell Biol 1992;10:2757-64.
21. Curran T, Franza BR. Fos and jun: the AP-1 connection. Cell 1988;55:395.
22. Janaswami PM, Kalvakolanu DV, Zhang Y, Sen GC. Transcriptional repression of the interleukin-6 gene by adenoviral protein E1A. J Biol Chem 1992;267:24886-91.
23. Grimm S, Baeuerle PA. The inducible transcription factor NF-κB: structure-function relationship of its protein subunits. Biochem J 1993;290:297-308.
24. Müller JM, Ziegler Heitbrock HWL, Baeuerle PA. Nuclear factor kappa B, a mediator of lipopolysaccharide effects. Immunobiol 1993;187:233-56.
25. Beg AA, Baldwin AS Jr. The IκB proteins: multifunctional regulators of Rel/NF-κB transcription factors. Genes Develop 1993;7:2064-70.
26. Cordle SR, Donald R, Read MA, Hawiger JJ. Lipopolysaccharide induces phos-

phorylationof MAD3 and activation of c-rel and related NF-κB proteins in human monocytic THP-1 cells. J Biol Chem 1993;268:11803-10.
27. Henkel T, Machleidt T, Alkalay I, Krönke M, Ben-Nerlah Y, Baeuerle PA. Rapid proteolysis of IκB-α is necessary for activation of transcription factor NF-κB. Nature 1993;365:182-85.
28. Ihle JN, Witthuhn BA, Quelle FW, et al. Signaling by the cytokine receptor superfamily: JAKs and STATs. Trends Biol Sci 1994;19:222-27.
29. Ihle JN, Kerr IM. JAKs and STATs in signaling by the cytokine receptor superfamily. Trends Genet 1995;11:69-74.
30. Darnell JE, Kerr IM, Stark GR. JAK/STAT pathways and transcriptional activation in response to IFNs and other extracellular signaling proteins. Science 1994;264:1415-21.
31. Nakajima K, Yamanaka Y, Nakae K, et al. A central role for Stat3 in IL-6-induced regulation of growth and differentiation in M1 leukemia cells. EMBO J 1996;15: 3651-58.
32. Finbloom DS, Winestock KD. IL-10 induces the tyrosine phosphorylation of Tyk2 and Jak1 and the differential assembly of STAT1 alpha and STAT3 complexes in human T cells and monocytes. J Immunol 1995;155:1079-90.
33. Tsukada J, Waterman WR, Koyama Y, Webb AC, Auron PE. A novel STAT-like factor mediates lipopolysaccharide, interleukin-1 (IL-1), and IL-6 signaling and recognizes a gamma interferon activation site-like element in the IL1ß gene. Mol Cell Biol 1996;16:2183-94.
34. Shuai K, Schindler C. Prezioso VR, Darnell JE. Activation of transcription by IFN-γ: tyrosine phosphorylation of a 91-kD DNA binding protein. Science 1992;259:1808-12.
35. Shuai K, Stark GR, Kerr IM, Darnell JE. A single phosphotyrosine residue Stat91 required for gene activation by interferon-γ. Science 1993;261:1744-46.
36. Hou J, Schindler U, Henzel WJ, Ho TC, Brasseur M, McKnight SL. An interleukin-4-induced transcription factor: IL-4 Stat. Science 1994;265:1701-6.
37. Marshall CJ. Specificity of receptor tyrosine kinase signaling: transient versus sustained extracellular signal-regulated kinase activation. Cell 1995;80:179-85.
38. Hunter T. Protein kinases and phosphatases: the Yin and Yang of protein phosphorylation and signaling. Cell 1995;80:225-36.
39. Nakajima T, Kinoshita S, Sasagawa T, et al. Phosphorylation at threonine-235 by a ras-dependent mitogen-activated protein kinase cascade is essential for transcription factor NF-IL6. Proc Natl Acad Sci 1993;90:2207-11
40. Gille H, Kortenjann M, Thomae O, et al. ERK phosphorylation potentiates Elk-1-mediated ternary complex formation and transactivation. EMBO J 1995;14:951-62.
41. Gupta S, Campbell D, Derijard B, Davis RJ. Transcription factor ATF-2 regulation by the JNK signal transduction pathway. Science 1995;267:389-93.
42. Van Dam H, Wilhelm D, Herr I, et al. ATF-2 is preferentially activated by stress-activated protein kinases to mediate c-jun induction in response to genotoxic agents. EMBO J 1995;14:1798-811.
43. Cavigelli M, Dolfi F, Claret F-X, Karin M. Induction of c-fos expression through JNK-mediated TCF-Elk-1 phosphorylation. EMBO J 1995;14:5957.

SIGNAL TRANSDUCTION FROM THE HAEMATOPOIETIC GROWTH FACTOR RECEPTORS

I.P. Touw[1]

Introduction

Haematopoietic growth factors (HGFs) act on the haematopoietic cells via binding to specific cell surface receptors. Many HGF receptors (HGF-R) have certain common structural features and have therefore been grouped in the superfamily of haematopoietin or cytokine receptors also referred to as the class I receptor superfamily [1,2]. Activation of these receptors by their respective HGFs is mediated through the formation of dimeric or oligomeric complexes of receptor structures. Some haematopoietin receptors are composed of heteromeric complexes, comprising two or three different receptor chains. For instance this is the case for receptors of interleukin IL-2, IL-3, IL-5, and granulocytemacrophage colony stimulating factor (GM-CSF) [3]. Other receptor structures, e.g., those of granulocyte--CSF (G-CSF) and erythropoietin (EPO), form homodimeric complexes upon growth factor binding [2,4]. This concise overview will start with an introduction to the basic principles of HGF-R signaling. Subsequently, a selection of the recent results obtained in this dynamic area of research, and their implications for our insights in the regulation of normal haematopoietic cell development as well as for understanding disease mechanisms will be briefly discussed.

Structural features of HGF receptors

Class I receptors are glycoproteins with an extracellular N-terminal domain, a single hydrophobic membrane spanning domain, and a C-terminal cytoplasmic domain. Characteristic of these receptors is the cytokine receptor homology (CRH) region in the extracellular domain that is required for HGF binding. The intracellular domains of class I receptors show little overall homology. Importantly, specific cellular responses to HGFs (e.g., proliferation and maturation), and the intracellular signaling mechanisms controlling them, are activated via distinct regions in the cytoplasmic domains of the receptors (Fig. 1).

1. I.P. Touw is supported by the Dutch Cancer Society and by a Pionier grant from N.W.O.

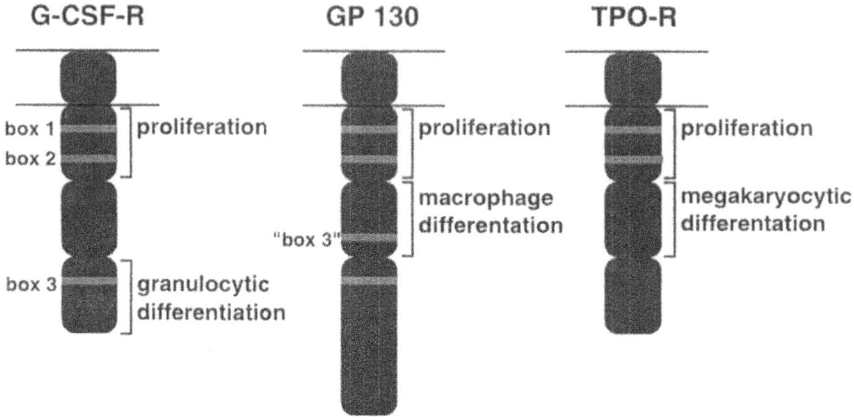

Figure 1. Schematic representation of the cytoplasmic domains of receptors for G-CSF, TPO and the IL-6 receptor signaling chain GP130. Signal transduction mechanisms involved in the induction of proliferation and maturation have been assigned to distinct subdomains of these receptors [5-7]. Boxes 1-3 represent stretches with weak structural homology [4].

Signal transduction

Phosphorylation of proteins on tyrosine (Tyr) or serine/threonine (Ser/Thr) residues, resulting in conformational changes, is a principle mechanism by which cytoplasmic signaling proteins can specifically interact and be activated as a consequence. Although the class I receptors activate cytoplasmic signaling substrates via tyrosine-phosphorylation, they do not possess tyrosine kinase activity themselves. Instead, protein tyrosine phosphorylation of downstream substrates is achieved via activation of cytoplasmic protein tyrosine kinases (PTKs). The Janus kinases (JAKs) comprise a PTK family with specific structural features that contains at least five members, four of which (JAKs 1-3, TYK2) have been found to play a central role in cytokine receptor signaling [8]. Activation of JAKs is essential for the mitogenic signaling function of HGF receptors. This became evident in experiments which showed that mutations in the membrane proximal

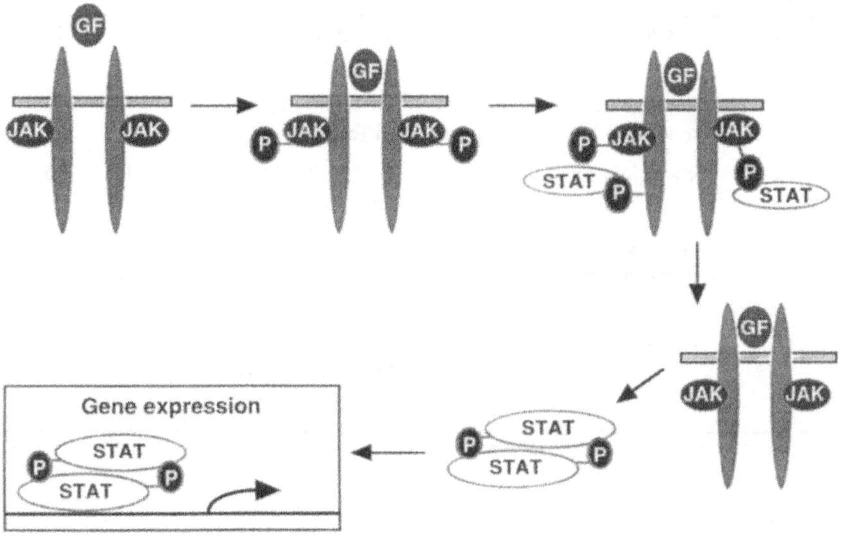

Figure 2. The JAK/STAT signaling pathway. Upon their phosphorylation on tyrosine (Y) residues by JAKs, STAT proteins form dimeric complexes. Note that binding of STATs to Y residues of the receptor protein may be required for recruitment and subsequent activation.

cytoplasmic region that prevent JAK-binding and activation completely abolish the proliferative signaling capacities of e.g., and GM-CSF-R and EPO-R [9,10]. In further support of this, overexpression of a kinase deficient form of JAK2 was found to interfere with EPO-induced proliferative responses [11]. Upon their activation, JAKs activate STAT (signal transducer and activator of transcription) proteins, which is generally seen as the major activity of the JAKs. However, as we will see later, this is not the only role that JAKs play in HGF-R signaling.

The JAK/STAT pathway is a very direct signaling pathway. Upon their activation, STAT proteins form complexes that immediately translocate to the nucleus, where they bind to specific transcription regulatory sequences in the genomic DNA and induce gene expression (Fig. 2). Thus far, 6 STAT proteins have been identified in mammalian cells, which activate distinct regulatory elements in the DNA. The HGF and cytokine receptors show characteristic STAT activation patterns, which raised the possibility that the diversity within the type of STAT complexes contributes to the nature of the cellular responses to a given cytokine/HGF [8]. Ample evidence in support of this comes from recent *in vivo* and *in vitro* studies in

Table 1. STATs and HGF/cytokine signaling: consequences of impaired STAT activity.

STAT type	Model	Affected HGF/cytokine response	Refs
STAT1	knock-out mice	IFN α and β; immunity to viral disease compromised	12, 13
STAT3	dominant negative mutants in murine leukemia cell line	IL-6; macrophage differentiation inhibited	14
STAT4	knock-out mice	IL-12; development of Th-1 and NK cells compromised	15, 16
STAT5	dominant negative mutants in murine cells	IL-3, GM-CSF, IL-5; proliferative signaling affected	17
STAT6	knock-out mice	IL-4; IgE class-switch blocked; development of Th-2 cells disturbed	18, 19

IFN= interferon; Th-1 = T-helper lymphocyte type 1; Th-2 = T-helper lymphocyte type 2; NK = natural killer cell.

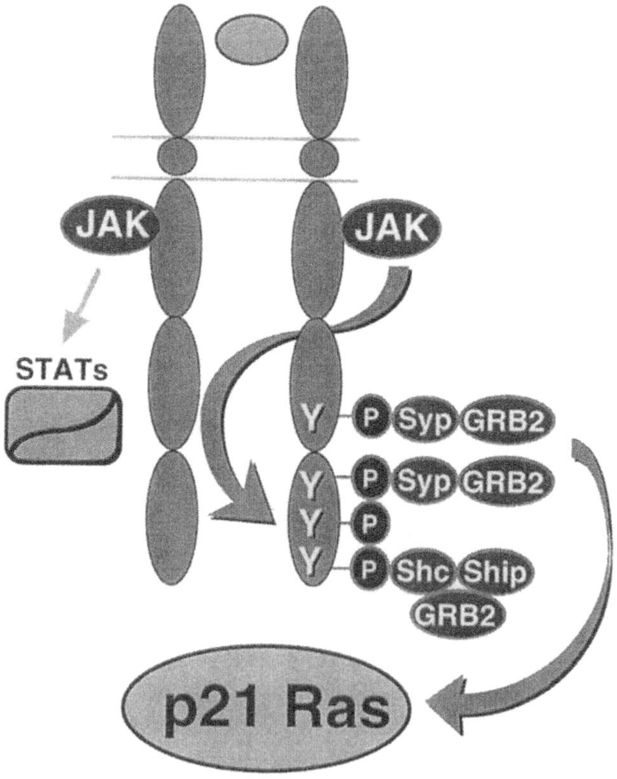

Figure 3. JAK kinases activate STATs, but are also required for cytokine receptor mediated activation of signaling molecules implicated in the p21Ras route [20].

Table 2. HGF-R defects and human disease.

Disease	Affected receptor	Mechanisms
X-linked SCID	IL-2, 7, 15-R γ chain	activation of JAK3 disturbed
Benign erythrocytosis	EPO-R	activation of HCP disturbed
Severe congenital neutropenia	G-CSF-R	defective maturation signaling
Acute myeloid leukemia	G-CSF-R	defective maturation signaling

See for text abbreviations and details.

which gene knockout or dominant negative mutant strategies were applied to specifically block the expression and/or function of STATs (Table 1).

A second major signaling mechanism activated by HGF-R involves the activation of p21Ras and the serine/threonine kinase MAPK. This route is more complex than the JAK/STAT pathway and can be activated via a variety of signaling intermediates, such as Shc/Grb2 and Syp/Grb2. The Ras/MAPK pathway is implicated in HGF supported survival of haematopoietic cells [3]. Further, signals given via the Ras route cooperate with JAK/STAT signals in controlling cell cycle progression. The co-operation between the JAK/STAT and Ras pathways is more intimate than was initially thought. Activation of the Ras route by, e.g., G-CSF-R cannot be achieved independent of JAKs [20]. This is because JAKs are (directly or indirectly) responsible for the phosphorylation of Tyr residues in the receptor molecules, which serve as binding sites for signaling substrates implicated in the p21Ras route (Fig. 3). Vice versa, although phosphorylation on tyrosine residues by JAKs suffices for STAT complex formation and DNA binding, it appeared that subsequent induction of transcription by STAT complexes requires an additional phosphorylation event, i.e., on serine residues [21]. This is achieved via members of the MAPK family, some of which are activated via the Ras signaling route [22] (Fig.4). Thus, "cross-talk" between the JAK/STAT and Ras/MAPK pathways may occur at least at two levels.

Abnormal receptor function in haematopoietic disorders

It has been envisaged that mutations in HGF receptor genes may have a role in certain haematopoietic diseases. In mice, it was shown that a mutation in the extracellular domain of EPO-R causes ligand independent activation of these receptors and leads to erythroleukemia [23]. Such transforming mutations have, as yet, not been identified in clinical leukemias. Structural abnormalities might also result in impaired function of the cytoplasmic domains of HGF receptors. Until now, such defects have been found in four human haematologic disorders: X-linked severe combined immunodeficiency (X-SCID); benign erythrocytosis, also known as primary familial and congenital polycythemia; severe congenital neutropenia (SCN) and acute myeloblastic leukemia (AML) (Table 2).

X-SCID is a congenital disease characterized by severely hampered function of

B cells and a complete deficiency of T-cells. Responses to multiple cytokines involved in B and T cell development, particularly IL-2, IL-7 and IL-15, are impaired in these patients. The gene encoding the common receptor chain (γ_c) of these cytokines is located on the X-chromosome. Several point mutations, resulting in the truncation of the cytoplasmic domain of the γ_c protein, have been found in X-SCID [24]. These truncations abrogate the mitogenic signaling function of the IL-2R, IL-7R and IL-15R complexes. Two independent lines of evidence indicate that the inability of the truncated γ_c proteins to activate JAK3 plays a central role in this defect. First, knock-out mice lacking the JAK3 gene have symptoms very similar to SCID [25]. Second, a patient with mutations in the JAK3 gene leading to a complete lack of JAK3 expression, experienced clinical symptoms very similar to those of X-SCID patients [26].

Benign erythrocytosis is a dominant condition characterized by a mild increase in red blood cell counts with normal serum levels of EPO. Point mutations in the EPO-R, resulting in the truncation of approximately 70 C-terminal amino acids of the EPO-R were originally found in a large Finnish family, but have subsequently been identified in individuals from several other families [27,28]. These mutations delete a subdomain that is involved in the binding of a protein tyrosine phosphatase haematopoietic cell phosphatase (HCP). Because HCP is a negative regulator of JAK activation, the mitogenic responses to EPO are enhanced in these patients [29].

Severe congenital neutropenia (SCN) is a group of haematopoietic disorders characterized by profound absolute neutropenia and a maturation arrest of myeloid progenitor cells at the promyelocyte-myelocyte stage. As a result, patients suffer

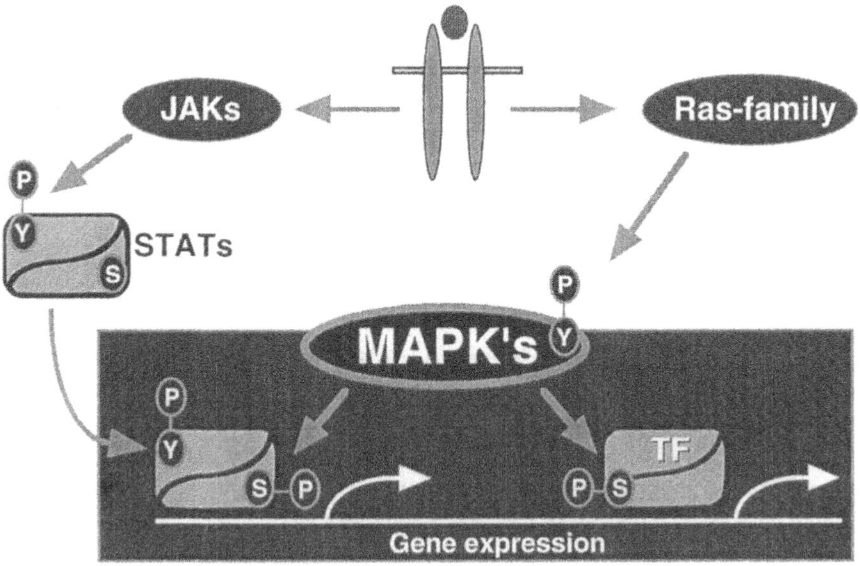

Figure 4. MAP kinases play a central role in activation of transcription factor complexes, including STAT complexes, via phosphorylation on serine (S) residues [21, 22].

from life threatening opportunistic infections. Some SCN patients have an increased susceptibility to myelodysplastic syndrome (MDS) or AML. Because defective G-CSF production and release of inhibitors of G-CSF could be excluded as common mechanisms causing neutropenia in SCN, it had been anticipated that G-CSF-R dysfunction might be involved in the pathogenesis of the disease.This idea gained support when a somatic mutation in the G-CSF-R gene was found in a case of SCN [30]. In a case of SCN [30]. This nonsense mutation resulted in the deletion of the C-terminal domain of G-CSF-R that has been functionally linked to maturation signaling. Given the fact that the truncated G-CSF-R protein, apart from lacking maturation signaling abilities, also misses the C-terminal element that negatively regulates proliferation, it was suggested that expression of this mutant receptor contributed to immortalization/enhanced self renewal capacity of myeloid progenitor cells. On this basis, the neutropenia in this case was believed to reflect a pre-leukemic condition. Indeed it could later be shown that the leukemic cells from AML patients with a history of SCN also had mutations in G-CSF-R, again truncating the C-terminal maturation-inducing region [31]. Significantly, G-CSF-R mutations that compromise the maturation signaling abilities of the receptor have also been detected in AML without a history of SCN, further supporting the notion that these types of mutations are oncogenic [32].

Acknowledgement

I am indebted to Karola van Rooyen for preparation of figures and slides. I thank my colleagues at the Institute of Haematology of the Erasmus University Rotterdam, especially John de Koning, Renée Barge and Bob Löwenberg, for discussions.

References

1. Bazan JF. Structural design and molecular evolution of a cytokine receptor superfamily. Proc Natl Acad Sci USA 1990;87:6934-38.
2. Cosman D. The haematopoietin receptor superfamily. Cytokine 1993;5:95-106.
3. Miyajima A, Mui ALF Ogorochi T, Sakamaki K. Receptors for granulocyte macrophage colony-stimulating factor, interleukin-3, and interleukin-5. Blood 1993;82: 1960-74.
4. Fukunaga R, Ishizaka-Ikeda E, Pan C-X, Seto Y Nagata S.Functional domains of the granulocyte colony-stimulating factor receptor. EMBO J 1991;10:2855-65.
5. Dong F, Van Buitenen C, Pouwels K, Hoefsloot LH, Löwenberg B, Touw IP. Distinct cytoplasmic regions of the granulocyte colony-stimulating factor receptor involved in induction of proliferation and maturation. Mol Cell Biol 1993;13:7774-81
6. Yamanaka Y Nakajima K, Fukada T, Hibi M, Hirano T. Differentiation and growth arrest signals are generated through the cytoplasmic region of gp130 that is essential for STAT3 activation. EMBO J 1996;15:1557-65.
7. Porteu F, Rouyez M-C, Cocault L, et al. Functional regions of the mouse thrombopoietin receptor cytoplasmic domain: Evidence for a critical region which is involved in differentiation and can be complemented by erythropoietin. Mol Cell Biol 1996; 16:2473-82.
8. Ihle JN, Kerr IM. JAKs and STATS in signaling by the cytokine receptor superfamily. Trends Genet 1995;11:69-74.

9. Quelle FW, Sato N, Witthuhn BA, et al. JAK2 associates with the β_c chain of the receptor for granulocyte-macrophage colony-stimulating factor, and its activation requires the membrane-proximal region. Mol Cell Biol 1994;14:4335-4.
10. Miura O, Cleveland JL, Ihle JN. Inactivation of erythropoietin receptor function by point mutations in a region having homology with other cytokine receptors. Mol Cell Biol 1993;13:1788-95.
11. Zhuang H, Patel SV, He T, Sonsteby S, Niu Z, Wojchowski DM. Inhibition of erythropoietin-induced mitogenesis by a kinase-deficient form of JAK2. J Biol Chem 1994;269:21411-14.
12. Meraz MA, White JM, Sheehan KCF, et al. Targeted disruption of the STAT1 gene in mice reveals unexpected physiologic specificity in the JAK-STAT signaling pathway. Cell 1996;84:431-42.
13. Durbin JE, Hackenmiller R, Simon MC, Levy DE. Targeted disruption of the mouse STAT1 gene results in compromised innate immunity to viral disease. Cell 1996;85: 443-50.
14. Nakajima K, Yamanaka Y, Nakae K, et al. A central role for STAT3 in IL-6-induced regulation of growth and differentiation in M1 leukemia cells. EMBO J 1996;15: 3651-58.
15. Thierfelder WE, van Deursen JM, Yamamoto K, et al. Requirement for STAT4 in interleukin-12 mediated responses of natural killer cells. Nature 1996;382:171-74.
16. Kaplan MH, Sun Y-L, Hoey T, Grusby MJ. Impaired IL-I2 responses and enhanced development of Th cells in STAT-4-deficient mice. Nature 1996;382:174-77.
17. Mui ALF, Wakao H, O'Farrell AM, Harada N, Miyajima A. Interleukin-3, granulocyte macrophage colony stimulating factor and interleukin-5 transduce signals through two STAT5 homologs. EMBO J 1995;14:1166-75.
18 Takeda K, Tanaka T, Shi W, et al .Essential role of STAT6 in IL-4 signaling. Nature 1996;380:627-30.
19. Shimoda K, van Deursen J, Sangster MY, et al. Lack of IL-4-induced Th2 response and IgE class switching in mice with disrupted STAT6 gene. Nature 1996;380: 630-33.
20. Barge RMY, de Koning JP, Pouwels K, Dong F, Löwenberg B, Touw IP. Tryptophan 650 of human granulocyte colony-stimulating factor (G-CSF) receptor, implicated in the activation of JAK2, is also required for G-CSF-mediated activation of signaling complexes of the p21Ras route. Blood 1996;87:2148-53.
21. Wen Z, Zhong Z, Darnell JE. Maximal activation of transcription by STAT1 and STAT3 requires both tyrosine and serine phosphorylation. Cell 1995;82:241-50.
22. David M, Petricoin III E, Benjamin C, Pine R, Weber MJ, Larner A-C. Requirement for MAP kinase (ERK2) activity in interferon α- and interferon β-stimulated gene expression through STAT proteins. Science 1995;269: 1721-23.
23. Longmore GD, Lodish HF. An activating mutation in the murine erythropoietin receptor induces erythroleukemia in mice: A cytokine receptor superfamily oncogene. Cell 1991;67: 1089-102.
24. Noguchi M, Yi H, Rosenblatt HM, et al. Interleukin-2 receptor γ chain mutation results in X-linked severe combined immunodeficiency in humans. Cell 1993;73: 147-57.
25. Nosaka T, van Deursen JMA, Tripp, et al. Defective lymphoid development in mice lacking JAK3. Science 1995;270:800-2.
26. Russell SM, Tayebi N, Nakajima H, et al. Mutation of JAK3 in a patient with SCID: Essential role of JAK3 in lymphoid development. Science 1995;270:797-800.
27. De la Chapelle A, Träskelin AL, Juvonen E. Truncated erythropoietin receptor causes dominantly inherited benign human erythrocytosis. Proc Natl Acad Sci USA 1993;90: 4495-99.
28. Sokol L, Luhovy M, Guan y, Prchal JF, Semenza GL, Prchal JT. Primary familial poly-

cythemia: A frameshift mutation in the erythropoietin receptor gene and increased sensitivity of erythroid progenitors to erythropoietin. Blood 1995;86: 15-22.

29. Klingmüller U, Lorenz U, Cantley LC, Neel BG, Lodish HF. Specific recruitment of SH-PTP 1 to the erythropoietin receptor causes inactivation of JAK2 and termination of proliferative signals. Cell 1995;80:729-38.
30. Dong F, Hoefsloot LH, Schelen AM, et al. Identification of a nonsense mutation in the granulocyte colony-stimulating factor receptor in severe congenital neutropenia. Proc Natl Acad Sci USA 1994;91:4480-84.
31. Dong F, Brynes RK, Tidow N, Welte K, Löwenberg B, Touw IP. Mutations truncating the C-terminal maturation region of the G-CSF receptor in acute myeloid leukemia preceded by severe congenital neutropenia. N Engl J Med 1995;333: 487-93.
32. Dong F, van Paassen M, van Buitenen C, Hoefsloot LH, Löwenberg B, Touw IP. A point mutation in the granulocyte colony-stimulating factor receptor (G-CSF-R) gene in a case of acute myeloid leukemia results in the overexpression of a novel G-CSF-R isoform. Blood 1995;85:902-11.

RECIPIENT IMMUNE RESPONSES INDUCED BY ALLOGENEIC WHOLE BLOOD OR PLATELET TRANSFUSIONS: IMPLICATIONS FOR IMMUNOMODULATION[1]

J.W. Semple, D. Cosgrave, E.R. Speck, A. Bang, V.S. Blanchette, J. Freedman

Introduction

CD4+ T helper (Th) cell responses can be divided in Th0, Thl and Th2 [l-4]. These responses are categorized based on the identification of cytokines. Th1-like responses generally produce interleukin (IL)-2/interferon-γ (IFN-γ), primarily mediate cell mediated immunity and, in mice, induce the synthesis of IgG_{2a} antibodies whereas Th2-like responses on the other hand generally produce IL-4, IL-5, IL-6 and IL-l0 and are superior at inducing IgG_1 and IgE humoral immunity [1-4]. Th0-like responses are thought to be less differentiated than those mediating Thl and Th2 responses because cytokines characteristic of both e.g. IL-4, IFN-γ and IL-10, etc. can be identified. What makes these patterns of cytokines so intriguing is that they appear to be associated with different immune functions. With respect to transplantation, for example, there is compelling evidence that Thl responses are associated with graft rejection [5-9], whereas Th2 responses may be correlated with immune tolerance towards the graft [10-13].

In both human and animal studies, several reports have demonstrated that whole blood (WB) transfusions induce recipient immunosuppressive effects; the so-called transfusion effect [l4-19]. The mechanism(s) mediating this phenomenon are unknown, but Dallman et al. [20] have demonstrated reduced production of IL-2 and expression of the IL-2 receptor in whole blood (WB) transfusion recipients, suggesting an IL-2 defect whereas Babcock et al. [21] have shown that WB transfusions induce *in vitro* Th2 cytokine profiles in mice. Similar results have also been found in human recipients of WB [22]. These cytokine results may have relevance to the role that WB transfusions play in non-responsiveness to alloantigens.

There is controversy as to whether platelets can mediate the transfusion effect [23-26]. Using a murine model, we have demonstrated that leukoreduced allogeneic platelet transfusions stimulate *in vitro* recipient CD4+ Th1 cellular responses mediated by indirect allorecognition [27]. Indirect allorecognition occurs when donor-derived antigens are processed and presented by recipient antigen presenting cells (APC) to recipient Th cells which ultimately stimulate anti-donor antibody synthesis. This mechanism of platelet-induced alloimmunity was confirmed by Oh

1. This work was supported by a grant (TO.02.95) from the Canadian Red Cross Blood Services.

et al. [28] who found that recipient adherent macrophages were responsible for inducing humoral immunity against allogeneic platelets in inbred rats.

Collectively, these data suggest that allogeneic platelets may stimulate a qualitatively different recipient immune response compared with transfusions of WB which may have a role in recipient immunomodulation. We have compared the immunoglobulin isotype of anti-donor antibodies and Th cytokine responses induced by either allogeneic WB or platelet transfusions. In healthy recipients, WB transfusions stimulate polarized Th2-like immune responses, whereas allogeneic platelets are associated with a strong Th1-like response.

Materials and methods

Animals and cell lines

Female BALB/c (H-2^d) mice, 8-12 wks of age were used as the transfusion recipients and female C57BL/6 (H-2^b) mice, 6-10 wks of age were used as platelet donors; the mice were purchased from Harlan-Sprague Dawley (Indianapolis, IN). The cell lines, P815 (H-2^d) mastocytoma, EL-4 (H-2^b) thymoma and R1.1 (H-2^k) lymphoma were used as MHC typing cells and were purchased from the ATCC (Rockville, MD). All the cell lines and *in vitro* assays were maintained in RPMI-1640 with 5% fetal calf serum (FCS), 100 μg/ml Penicillin/Streptomycin/Fungizone, 100 mM L-glutamine and 5×10^{-5} M 2-mercaptoethanol.

Cell preparation and transfusion protocol

For whole blood, mice were bled via the tail vein into EDTA-microvettes (Starstedt, St. Laurent, Que) filled with 5 μl sodium heparin. Platelets were prepared as previously described [27]. Briefly, whole blood was pooled, centrifuged at 120×g, and the platelet rich plasma (PRP) aspirated off; care was taken not to disturb or aspirate the buffy coat. The platelets were washed 3× in 1% EDTA-saline and 'contaminating' leukocytes were enumerated by a Nageotte haemocytometer (Baxter, Chicago, IL) and by flow cytometry as previously described [27,29]. Using these methods we can detect ≤ 0.5 WBC/μl. For these studies, the mean leukocyte contamination in the platelets transfused was 1.6±1.4 WBC/μl. For spleen cells, mice were sacrificed, spleens removed and teased into single cell suspensions. The cells were layered on a 1.077 g/ml Percoll cushion and cells enriched by centrifugation at 1800×g for 30 min at 20°C.

For transfusion, platelets were adjusted to 2×10^9 cells/ml. In each transfusion protocol, all mice were pre-bled 24 h prior to the first transfusion and then injected (100 μl) with either platelets or whole blood weekly via the tail vein. Mice were bled weekly for sera and at day 7 post-transfusion (PT), a group of 10 mice were sacrificed for spleen cells. Ten control non-transfused mice were assayed at each time interval.

ConA cultures

In vitro cytokine production from recipient spleen cells was assessed in 48 h Concanavalin A (ConA) cultures using 1 μg of ConA (Sigma) as previously de-

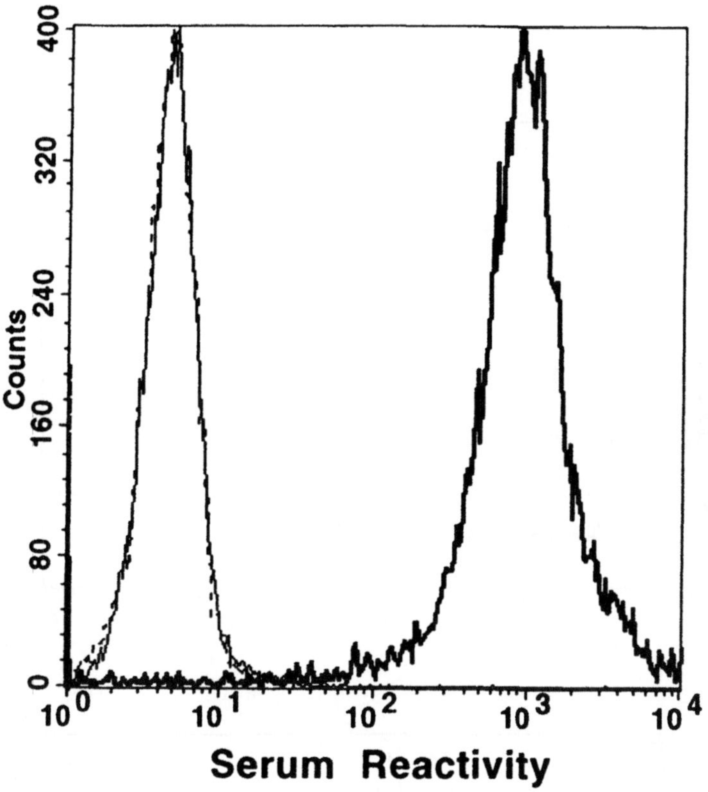

Figure 1. Flow cytometric analysis of anti-MHC specificity in sera from mice transfused with platelets at week 5 PT. EL-4 (H-2^b) (——), P815 (H-2^d) (-------) or R1.1 (H-2^k) (——) cell lines were incubated with a 1/25 dilution of recipient serum and labelled with FITC-GAM IgG. Results were similar for mice transfused with WB.

scribed [27]. Briefly, 10^5 recipient spleen cells were incubated with the mitogen in 300 µ l triplicate cultures for 48 h at 37°C and 200 µl of supernatants were removed and frozen at -80°C for cytokine determinations.

Sera preparation and cytokine determinations

Blood was allowed to clot for 1 h on ice and centrifuged at 3,000×g at 4°C. The sera were collected and frozen at -80°C. All sera were analyzed for the presence of IL-4, IL-10 and interferon-γ by commercial ELISA's (Immunocorp, Montreal, Que). Standard curves were generated with titrations of recombinant cytokines.

Flow cytometric analyses of sera

For detection of recipient IgG anti-donor antibodies, 10^5 donor or recipient WBC were incubated with dilutions of recipient sera for 45 min at 20°C, washed 1× and labeled with FITC-conjugated goat anti-mouse (FITC-GAM) IgG (Fc specific, Cedarlane Laboratories, Hornby, Ont) for 30 min at 20°C in the dark. For Th1 or Th2 dominated immunoglobulin subclasses [30], cells were labeled with

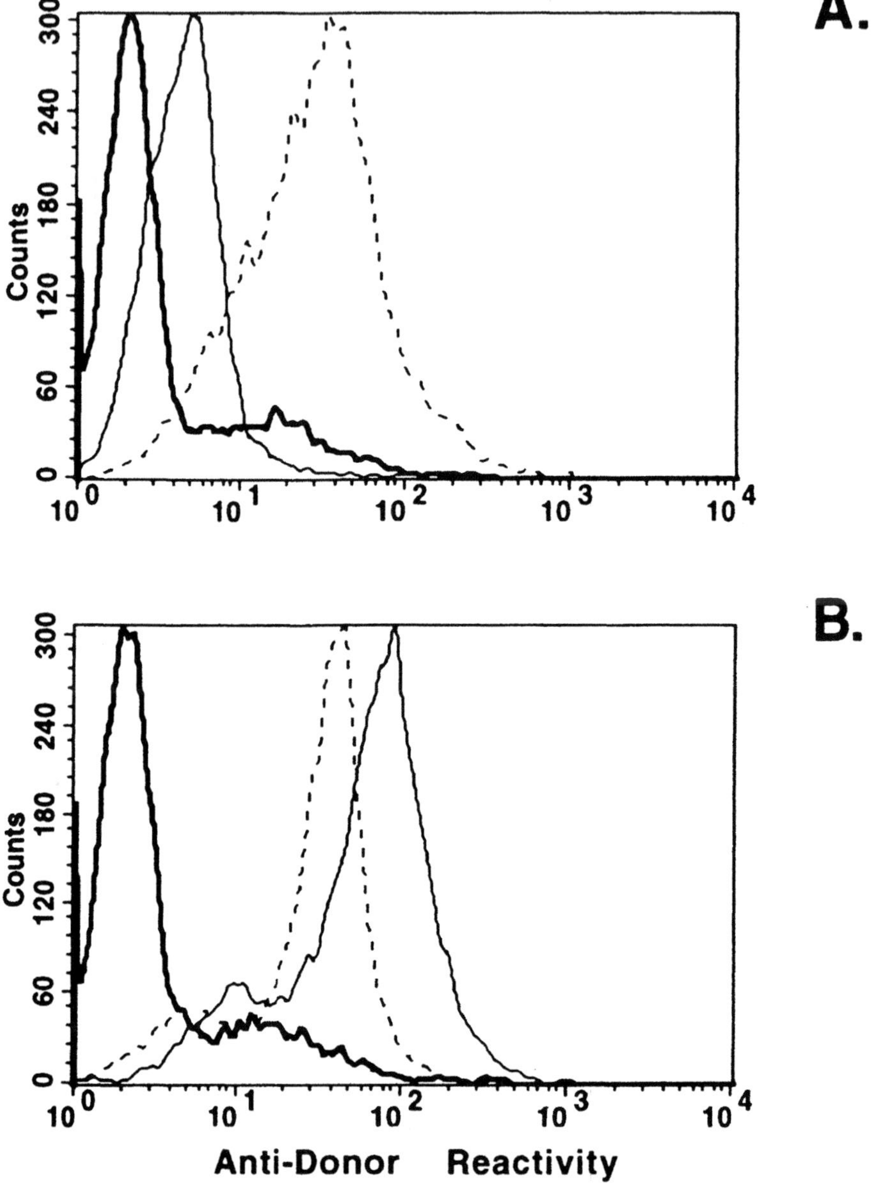

Figure 2. Flow cytometric analysis of IgG anti-donor isotypes in recipient sera from mice transfused with either (A) WB (week 2 PT) or (B) platelets (week 5 PT). Donor (C57BL/6) spleen cells were incubated with a 1/25 dilution of recipient serum and labeled with FITC-GAM IgG_1 (------) or IgG_{2a} (——). Prebleed serum (——) was used as the negative control.

Table 1. Day 7 post-transfusion cytokine levels (pg/ml) in the sera of mice (N=10) transfused with either platelets or WB.

	Non-transfused	**Platelet transfused**	**WB transfused**
IL-4	N.D.	N.D.	95±26
IL-10	N.D.	N.D.	29±8
IFN-γ	N.D.	22±5	N.D.

N.D. = Not detected (ELISA sensitivities were: IL-4 >31.3 pg/ml; IL-10 >15.6 pg/ml; IFN-γ,>15.6 pg/ml). Data is presented as mean pg/ml ± SD.

either FITC-GAM IgG_{2a} (Cedarlane) or FITC-GAM IgG_1 (Cedarlane) respectively. Cells were analyzed on a FACSort flow cytometer (Becton Dickinson, San Jose, CA) operating with an argon ion laser at 15 mW; 10,000 events were acquired using an electronic cellular gate based on forward and side scatter and were analyzed using LYSYS II software (Becton Dickinson). Matched pre-bleed serum was used as the negative control in all experiments. Donor specificity of the IgG was confirmed by positive reactivity with EL-4 (H-2^b) cells but absence of reactivity with P815 (H-2^d) [24] or third party R1.1 cells (H-2^k).

Statistical methods

Significance between means was determined by Student's t test.

Results

Anti-donor antibody responses induced by WB or platelet transfusions

To characterize anti-donor antibodies produced by WB or platelet transfusions, recipient sera were analyzed by flow cytometry. Control transfusions (upto 10) with syngeneic WB or platelets did not induce IgG anti-donor responses in any mice tested (N=20). In contrast, allogeneic WB transfusions induced IgG anti-donor antibody formation in all recipient mice by the second transfusion whereas platelet transfusions induced alloantibodies by the fifth transfusion. Titres of the IgG alloantibodies ranged from 1:1,024-4,096 for WB transfusions and 1:256-4,096 for platelet transfusions. The sera reacted with cells expressing donor MHC (H-2^b) but not with cells expressing recipient (H-2^d) or third party MHC (H-2^k) (Fig. 1). Characterization of Th1-mediated IgG_{2a} and Th2-mediated IgG_1 isotypes showed that WB transfusions induced the production of primarily IgG_1 anti-donor antibodies (Fig. 2A). In contrast, platelet transfusions stimulated a significant IgG_{2a} anti-donor antibody response together with IgG_1 anti-donor antibodies (Fig. 2B).

In vivo and *in vitro* cytokine responses generated by platelet or whole blood transfusions

To determine the effects that platelet or WB transfusions have on recipient *in vivo* Th cytokine patterns, sera were analyzed by ELISA before and at day 7 post-transfusion (PT). Prebleed sera had undetectable levels of IL-4, IL-10 and

Table 2. Cytokine levels (pg/ml) in ConA-stimulated spleen cell cultures from mice (N=10) transfused with either platelets or WB

	Non-transfused	Platelet transfused[1)]	WB transfused[1)]
IL-4	540±58	148±62	968±279
IL-10	170±83	625±311	1,010±273
IFN-γ	57±15	267±51	86±29

1. Mice were sacrificed and tested at day 7 PT. Data is presented as mean pg/ml ± SD.

IFN-γ. WB transfusions, by day 7 PT, caused a significant increase in serum levels of IL-4 and IL-10 but not IFN-γ (Table 1) whereas mice receiving platelet transfusions had detectable levels of IFN-γ at day 7 PT but not IL-4 or IL-10 (Table 1).

To demonstrate that the *in vivo* produced cytokines were produced by T cells, supernatants from ConA-stimulated spleen cell cultures were analyzed. Cytokine levels in ConA cultures from non-transfused control mice were; IL-4: 540 pg/ml, IL-10: 170 pg/ml and IFN-γ: 57 pg/ml and these cytokines were detected in all the culture supernatants. By comparison, spleen cells from WB recipients at day 7 PT secreted significantly higher levels of IL-4 (968 pg/ml) whereas IFN-γ levels were not significantly changed (86 pg/ml). In contrast, IL-4 production in the ConA cultures of platelet recipients was significantly reduced (148 pg/ml) and IFN-γ production was increased (267 pg/ ml) (Table 2). IL-10 production, on the other hand was increased in the ConA cultures from both platelet and WB recipients (625 and 1,010 pg/ml respectively).

Thus, with respect to recipient anti-donor antibody and cytokine responses, platelet transfusions induce a significant Th1-mediated response whereas WB transfusions stimulate a predominantly Th2 response.

Discussion

There is increasing evidence which suggests that recipient Th1- and Th2-mediated immune responses can profoundly affect the outcome of a number of pathologic states e.g. resistance (Th1) or susceptibility (Th2) to parasitic infections [31] or allograft rejection and tolerance [5-13]. With respect to the latter, numerous animal and clinical studies have shown that pre-transplant donor specific WB transfusions correlate to increased graft survival [14-19] and recently, it has been shown that WB transfusions induce an *in vitro* Th2 cytokine profile [21]. It is still unclear however, what role the various cellular components of whole blood play in the recipient immune responses. We report a direct comparison of the anti-donor antibody isotypes and Th1/Th2 cytokine responses in recipients of either WB or leukoreduced platelet transfusions.

For many years, it has been suggested that leukoreduced allogeneic platelets are non-immunogenic with respect to MHC antigens. This speculation was primarily based on two early animal studies [22,33] which concluded that allogeneic platelets required leukocytes to stimulate recipient immune responses. Several laboratories, using flow cytometric techniques, have, however, more recently shown that even extreme leukoreduced allogeneic platelets are in fact immunogenic with respect to MHC molecules [27,34,35]. This result has also been found in a rat model of leukoreduced platelet transfusions (Dr. J.H. Oh, Department of Pathology, Emory University, Atlanta, GA., personal communication). Although these results would appear to have relevance to leukoreduction in human transfusions, it must be emphasized that as with all animal models, caution should be taken before extrapolating any data to the human situation. Nonetheless, there are many similarities with respect to immunity across mammalian species and fundamental transfusion-induced immune mechanisms may at least be identified. Furthermore, by studying healthy recipients, as can be done with animal models, the immune status of the recipient is more consistent so that the immunogenicity of transfusion can be validly addressed. In humans, recipients may be immunosuppressed e.g. due to cancer and/or chemotherapy, and this may have contributed to the belief that platelets are non-immunogenic with respect to the MHC.

In this study, we limited our definition of transfusion-induced alloimmunization to the identification of recipient IgG anti-donor alloantibodies. When recipients received allogeneic WB or platelet transfusions, both became alloimmunized although the time to alloimmunization and the immunoglobulin isotype of the anti-donor antibodies were different. WB transfusions induced predominantly IgG_1 anti-donor alloantibodies by the second transfusion whereas platelets induced significantly higher amounts of IgG_{2a} alloantibodies by the fifth transfusion. At first, these data would appear to suggest that WB transfusions are more immunogenic than platelets (2 weeks to antibody production for WB compared with 5 weeks for platelets). However, once alloantibodies were induced by the platelet transfusions, their titres were comparable with those stimulated by WB. Additionally, we do not believe that the trace numbers of contaminating leukocytes ($\approx$ 1.6 cells/μl) within the platelets were responsible for any of the IgG synthesis since it has been shown that this number is approximately 10-fold below the immunogenic threshold for weekly allogeneic leukocyte transfusions to stimulate anti-donor antibodies [27,33].

Based on the immunoglobulin isotypes, the results support the concept that WB transfusions induce predominantly Th2-like IgG_1 anti-donor antibody responses whereas platelet transfusions have a strong Th1-like IgG_{2a} antibody component. These isotype responses may be related to the fundamental differences with which WB and platelets stimulate alloimmunity. Donor WB contains MHC class II positive antigen presenting cells (APC) which can directly activate recipient CD4+ T cells to initiate anti-donor alloimmune responses. Donor platelets on the other hand, because of their class I+/class II-MHC phenotype [27], cannot directly interact with recipient CD4+ T cells via MHC/T cell receptor interactions but first must be processed and presented by recipient MHC class II+ APC in order to activate Th cells [27,36]. These platelet-stimulated Th cells appear to have a strong Th1 cytokine profile which could significantly affect anti-donor antibody responses. In support of this, we have data which suggest that platelet-induced IgG_{2a} anti-donor responses are restricted to MHC class II I-A molecules on recipient macrophages [37]. Also of relevance are the recent findings of Gracie et al. [38] who demonstrated that MHC class I disparate WB transfusions between congenic and recombinant rat strains stimulate a strong Th1-mediated IgG_{2b}/IgG_{2c} response together with Th2-mediated IgG_1 anti-donor antibodies. Hence, the results support the basic concept that in allogeneic transfusion situations where the donor product has MHC class I disparities in the absence of class II molecules or disparities, recipients produce a strong Th1-mediated anti-donor response.

The Th cytokine responses in the recipient mice generally correlated with the alloantibody isotype analyses. By day 7 PT, *in vivo* Th2 like cytokine levels (IL-4 and IL-10) were seen in WB recipients whereas low but detectable levels of IFN-γ was found in the sera of platelet recipients and the *in vitro* (ConA) cytokine responses confirmed these results. Additionally, our *in vitro* data supports the previous observations of Babcock et al. [21] indicating Th2-like cytokine production in WB recipients. Thus, these *in vivo* and *in vitro* cytokine patterns are consistent with the Th1-IgG_1 and Th2-IgG_{2a} anti-donor isotypes present in the WB and platelet recipients respectively. Although it is not clear how the platelet transfusions also stimulated IgG_1 production in the apparent absence of *in vivo* IL-4 and IL-10, the presence of increased IL-10 together with smaller amounts of IL-4 in the ConA cultures from platelet recipients suggests a Th2 component is active and may be responsible for generating the IgG_1 alloantibodies. Alternatively, IgG_1 production induced by allogeneic platelets may be independent of Th2-like cytokine patterns. This latter possibility may be related to our recent observations that platelet-induced IgG_1 and IgG_{2a} anti-donor responses are both dependent on the activation of induceable nitric oxide synthase within recipient macrophages [35].

Conclusions

Depending on the product transfused, recipient anti-donor alloimmune responses are significantly different with respect to alloantibody isotype and Th cytokine response. These alloimmune responses may be related to the observations that WB transfusions mediate the transfusion effect [14-19] whereas platelet transfusions may not [23-26]; WB-induced Th2 responses would be associated with allograft tolerance whereas platelet-induced Th1 responses may not mediate tolerance but would be more consistent with allograft rejection. We are currently studying this by analyzing donor skin graft survival in the immune recipients. What is most striking however, is that although it is clear that WB transfusions induce the transfusion effect [14-19], the recipients are by definition (IgG) also highly alloimmunized against the donors MHC haplotype. We believe that transfusion-induced alloimmunization and immunosuppression are critically linked and analyzing both faces of this "double-edged sword" may be the key to understanding the mechanism(s) of recipient immune responses induced by various kinds of blood transfusions.

Acknowledgements

We would like to thank Drs. Alan Lazarus (St. Michael's Hospital) and Jung Oh (Emory University) for their helpful discussions.

References

1. Mosman TR, Cherwinski H, Bond MW, Giedlin MA, Coffman TL. Two types of mouse helper T cell clones: I. Definition according to profiles of lymphokine activities and secreted proteins. J Immunol 1986;136:2348-57.
2. Snapper CM, Paul WE. Interferon-γ and B cell stimulatory factor-1 reciprocally regulate Ig isotype production. Science 1986;236:944-47.
3. Cher D, Mosman TR. Two types of mouse helper T cell clones: II. Delayed-type hypersensitivity is mediated by Thl clones. J Immunol 1987;138:3688-94.
4. Mosman TR, Coffman RL. Thl and Th2 cells: different patterns of lymphokine secretion lead to different functional properties. Ann Rev Immunol 1989;7:145-73.
5. O'Connell P, Pacheco-Silva A, Nickerson P. Unmodified pancreatic islet allograft rejection results in the preferential expression of certain T cell activation transcripts. J Immunol 1993;150:1093-104.
6. Thai NL, Fu F, Qian S, et al. Cytokine mRNA profiles in mouse orthotopic liver transplantation. Graft rejection is associated with augmented Th1 function. Transplantation 1995;59:274-81.
7. Egawa H, Martinez OM, Quinn MB, et al. Acute liver allograft rejection in the rat. An analysis of the immune response. Transplantation 1995;59:97-102.
8. Takeuchi T, Lowry RP, Konieczny B. Heart allografts in mouse systems: the differential activation of Th2-like effector cells in peripheral tolerance. Transplantation 1992; 53:1281-94.
9. Hayashi M, Martinez OM, Garcia-Kennedy R, So S, Esquivel CO, Krams SM. Expression of cytokines and immune mediators during chronic liver allograft rejection. Transplantation 1995;60:1533-38.
10. Landorfo S, Cofano F, Giovarelli, Prat M, Cavallo G, Forni G. Inhibition of interferon-gamma may suppress allograft reactivity by T lymphocytes *in vitro* and *in vivo*. Science 1985;229:176-79.
11. Chen N, Field EH. Enhanced type 2 and diminished type 1 cytokines in neonatal tolerance. Transplantation 1995;59:933-41.
12. Mottram PL Han W-R, Purcell LJ, McKenzie IFC Hancock WW. Increased expression of IL-4 and IL-10 and decreased expression of IL-2 and interferon-γ in long-surviving mouse heart allografts after brief CD4-monoclonal antibody therapy. Transplantation 1995;59:559-65.
13. Donckier V, Wissing M, Bruyns C, et al. Critical role of interleukin 4 in the induction of neonatal transplantation tolerance. Transplantation 1995;59:1571-76.
14. Opelz G, Senger DPS, Mickey MR, Terasaki PI. Effect of blood transfusions on subsequent kidney transplants. Transplant Proc 1973;5:253 -55.
15. Fabre JW, Bishop M, SenT, et al. A study of three protocols of blood transfusion before renal transplantation in the dogs. Transplantation 1978;26:94-98.
16. Quigley RL, Wood KJ, Morris PJ. Investigation of the mechanism of active enhancement of renal allograft survival by blood transfusion. Immunol 1988;163:373-81.
17. Soulillou J-P, Blandin F, Gunther E, Lemoine V. Genetics of the blood transfusion effect on heart allografts in rats. Transplantation 1984;38:63-67.
18. Shirwan H, Wang HK, Barwari L, Makowka L, Cramer DV. Pretransplant injection of allograft recipients with donor blood or lymphocytes permits allograft tolerance without the presence of persistent donor chimerism. Transplantation 1996;61:1382-86.

19. Wood PJ, Roberts ISD, Yang C-P, Cossens IA, Bell ER. Prevention of chronic rejection by donor-specific blood transfusion in a new model of chronic cardiac allograft rejection. Transplantation 1996;61:1440-43.
20. Dallman MJ, Shiho O, Page TH, Wood KJ, Morris PJ. Peripheral tolerance to alloantigen results from altered regulation of the interleukin-2 pathway. J Exp Med 1991;173: 79-87.
21. Babcock GF, Alexander JW. The effects of blood transfusion on cytokine production by Th1 and Th2 lymphocytes in the mouse. Transplantation 1996;61:465-68.
22. Kalechman Y, Gafter U, Sobelman D, Sredni B. The effect of a single whole-blood transfusion on cytokine secretion. J Clin Immunol 1990;10:99-105.
23. Chapman JR, Ting A, Fisher M. Failure of platelet transfusion to improve human renal allograft survival. Transplantation 1986;41:468-73.
24. Bijnen AB, Heineman E, Marquet RL, et al. Lack of beneficial effect of thrombocyte transfusions on the kidney graft survival in dogs. Transplantation 1984;37:213-14.
25. Oh JH, McClure HM, Tuttle EP. Immunological unresponsiveness induced by platelet transfusions in rhesus monkeys. Transplantation 1983;36:727-28.
26. Hibberd AD, Scott LJ. Allogeneic platelets increase the survival of rat renal allografts. Transplantation 1983;35:622-24.
27. Semple JW, Speck ER, Milev YP, Blanchette V, Freedman J. Indirect allorecognition of platelets by T helper cells during platelet transfusions correlates with anti-MHC antibody and cytotoxic T lymphocyte formation. Blood 1995;86:805-12.
28. Oh JH, Taysavang P, Whelchel JD. Conferring immunogenicity to platelets by preincubation with recipients' adherent cells. Proc IX International Congress of Immunology. San Francisco, CA, 1995;p 69 (Abstr).
29. Kao KJ, Scornik JC. Accurate quantitation of the low number of white cells in white cell-depleted blood components. Transfusion 1989;29:774-77.
30. Finkelman FD, Holmes J, Katona IM, et al. Lymphokine control of *in vivo* immunoglobulin isotype selection. Ann Rev Immunol 1990;8:303-33.
31. Sher A, Coffman RL. Regulation of immunity to parasites by T cells and T cell-derived cytokines. Ann Rev Immunol 1992;10:385-409.
32. Welsh KI, Burgos H, Batchelor JR. The immune response to allogeneic rat platelets; Ag-B antigens in matrix form lacking Ia. Eur J Immunol 1977;7:267-72.
33. Claas FHJ, Smeenk RJT, Schmidt R, Van Steenbrugge GJ, Eernisse JG. Alloimmunization against the MHC antigens after platelet transfusions is due to contaminating leukocytes in the platelet suspension. Exp Hematol 1981;9:84-89.
34. Kao KJ. Effects of leukocyte depletion and UVB irradiation on alloantigenicity of major histocompatibility complex antigens in platelet concentrates: A comparative study. Blood 1992;80:2931-37.
35. Bang A, Speck ER, Blanchette VS, Freedman J, Semple JW. Recipient humoral immunity against leukoreduced allogeneic platelets is suppressed by aminoguanidine, a selective inhibitor of inducible nitric oxide synthase (iNOS). Blood 1996;88:2959-66.
36. Bang A, Hicks KJ, Speck ER, Blanchette V, Freedman J, Semple JW. Allogeneic platelets require unique antigen processing mechanisms within recipient antigen presenting cells (APC) in order to stimulate alloantibody production. Blood, 1996; 88(Suppl 1): 162a.
37. Semple JW, Speck ER, Blanchette V, Freedman J. Immune non-responsiveness to allogeneic platelets in murine strains which lack MHC class II I-E molecules is due to the presence of CD8+ T cells. Blood, 1996;88 (Suppl 1):162a.
38. Gracie JA, Bradley JA: Interleukin-12 induces interferon-γ-dependent switching of IgG alloantibody subclass. Eur J Immunol, 1996;26:1217-21.

DISCUSSION

B. Löwenberg and C.Th. Smit Sibinga – moderators

B. Löwenberg (Rotterdam, NL): Dr. Spits, in fact you showed two sets of data to indicate the relationship between the induction of T-cell receptor arrangement and IL-7; one was the in vitro data in the foetal liver, the subset of CD34 negative foetal liver cells where you could induce T-cell re-arrangement and then the knock out that was a negative experiment. Does this imply that the in vitro experiment was not a pure experiment, because perhaps there was a minor subset of cells that already were rearranged in that expanded subset.

H. Spits, (Amsterdam, NL): Of course, the in vitro experiment and the interpretations of these in vitro experiments were hampered by the fact that this type of experiment was done with bulk cultures of cells. On the other hand, perhaps there is something different between the mouse and human. In the human X-linked SCID, there is a real mutation which has a complete non-functional gamma chain, there are no T-cells at all. Also in the time, if you find accumulation you find receptor rearrangements that are accumulated in the DJ re-arrangement so you have no VDJ re-arrangement. We have found that if you take the cell population that has DJ rearrangement but not VD arrangement, and culture it out in IL-7 than you get VDJ re-arrangements. So it remains difficult, but it can also point to a fundamental difference between mouse and man and the requirements for an intact gamma chain.

L.T. Goudnough (St. Louis, MO, USA): Dr. Semple, actually a two-part question on the clinical effect of this immunomodulation; the first part is a question with respect to whole blood transfusion. As you know the so-called immunosuppressive effect from whole blood is controversial with respect to post-operative infections or cancer recurrence and I would agree with you that as far as I am concerned the most compelling evidence would be in the renal allograft experience. Even in the original description by Opelz and Terasaki[1], when they looked at the effect of previous transfusions on subsequent one year survival of the renal allograft it was clearly there, but there was also a table of a cohort of patients who had never been previously transfused but who were transfused at the time of the kidney transplant. When they looked at the one year allograft survival in that cohort there was no

1. Opelz G, Terasaki PI. Enhancement of kidney graft survival by blood transfusion. Transplant Proc 1977;9:121-22.

difference compared to those, who had never been previously transfused and also were untransfused at the time of the renal allograft. So, I am uncertain even there. If we want to have a paradigm of the risk of transfusions on subsequent allograft survival or post operative infections or cancer recurrence, I remain to be convinced that there is a defined clinical effect for whole blood. The second part of the comment or question is with respect to platelets. You seem to imply that the TRAP study report in 1996 is somehow going to have a comment about the clinical effect and I was wondering if you are going to share some of those results with us.

J.W. Semple (Toronto, C): Well in the first part in terms of whole blood I agree with you; I do not think that whole blood is as immunosuppressive as the literature may suggest and in fact from our data these mice are alloimmunised by the definition of alloimmunisation being anti-donor IgG. I believe that it is the type of T-cell response which determines outcome; Th1 tends to be associated with graft rejection whereas Th2 responses tend to be associated with graft tolerance. It may very well be that these mice are not immuno-suppressed at all. In fact they simply make an immune response in a qualitatively different way. The Th2 cytokines in that milieu allow the graft possibly to survive, but I agree totally in terms of the clinical situation; I do not believe the results are really all that compelling for true immunosuppression.

Now the second question, the TRAP study. It is clear from all the small clinical studies that have taken place both in the US and in Europe, that leukoreduction reduces alloimmunisation. You have to come back and think about the recipient. These recipients are cancer patients; leukaemics. Primarily, they have been on chemotherapy at some point during the transfusion protocol and so they have an immune system that we know is abnormal. So, this indirect system that I am talking about with respect to platelets is sensitive to immunosuppression. It may be that these leukaemics have simply lost this mechanism, because we know that leuko-reduction tends to reduce alloimmunisation to platelets. The TRAP study is going to be presented at the AABB[1] and Dr. Schiffer will give those results.

H. Spits: Dr. Semple, do you have any direct evidence that the Th2 cells you get are alloreactive cells. The second question: is there any indication that also in humans you have something like this, because in human it is much more difficult to induce these polarised Th1, Th2 potencies than in mice.

J.W. Semple: In humans it is zero. If you look at most of the literature in humans it is mostly Th0. In terms of the first question, we have been looking at skin graft survivals in the whole blood recipients and in mice that had spleen cells transferred from the whole blood recipients. The results are preliminary, but suggest that in fact

---

1. Reducing alloimmunisation: results of new clinical studies. Schiffer ChA. Results of the American 'TRAP' study. Scientific short seminar, 49th annual meeting of the AABB, Orlando, FL, October 14,1996.

the transferred mice may have a prolonged skingraft survival. However, these are preliminary results. We believe that we can transfer these Th2 responses to show an effect.

H. Spits: You would suggest that these Th2 cells are special cells?

J.W. Semple: I do not know if they are special, but the cytokines they produce certainly have a different effect than Th1. I do not think there is anything special about Th2 or Th1 cells. They are both CD4 positive and they both presumably have a similar α, β receptor. It depends on the antigen presenting cell and how the antigen is presented in the T-cells and it depends on the milieu that these T-cells are in at the time in terms of what is going to make them differentiate into 1, 2 or 0.

C.Th. Smit Sibinga (Groningen, NL): What has not been discussed and usually is avoided in the scientific approaches: is it the transfused circulating donor APC that continues producing cytokines that elicit the phenomenon or is it the passive transfusion of already produced cytokines in the transfusate that causes the phenomena?

E. Vellenga (Groningen, NL): When you look to the cytokine production in human beings and when you look especially to T-cells, one requirement for cytokine production by T-cells is that there has to be an activation of the T-cell receptor. This can be activated by CD3 or CD28, but the T-cell has to be activated before it can produce cytokines. I think that is the difference between cells belonging to the monocytic and granulocytic lineage; contact activation can induce cytokine expression. So I think it depends on the cytokine which you are studying. When you look at a specific cytokine produced by monocytic or granulocytic lineage, then I can believe that the processing of blood can result in cytokine production. I am not sure about T-cells because the activation of the T-cells and subsequently the expression of cytokines in T-cells is different. So, in some way IL-1 and IL-8 cannot be produced as a result of the ex vivo processing, but I am not sure about for example IL-4 or IL-5 or IL-2.

B. Löwenberg: Is there any direct evidence to indicate that for instance a platelet concentrate in a bag contains a significant amount of cytokines?

J.W. Semple: I think there is fairly good experimental data showing that a variety of different cytokines increase in platelet bags and it is thought, that most of the cytokines are produced from the contaminating leukocytes, for when you leukoreduce prestorage you will see less of those cytokines. However, plasma in the bag can in fact initiate a transfusion effect. I would not negate platelets themselves, because once they are leukoreduced, platelets are certainly full of pro-inflammatory cytokines and chemokines, which can evoke inflammatory-like responses.

B. Löwenberg: Dr. Spits, you discussed T-cell development and the important role of some selected cytokines for instance interleukin-7, a cytokine that induces expansion of some T-cells. Could you indicate your view on whether there would be a clinical applicability for producing selected types of T-cells taking advantage of this type of information?

H. Spits: Well, you undoubtedly know that in bone marrow transplantation and in particular in allogeneic bone marrow transplantation there are some problems with the development of the T-cell system. Although CD4 and CD8 positive cells can come back within 6 weeks after transplantation, these cells are not optimal and functional for a long time and that can be a problem for infections in these patients. So, perhaps it is a developmental problem that cytokines like IL-7 could be used in conditional therapy. After bone marrow transplantation you could give IL-7 to speed up or facilitate the development of T-cells. Concerning the use of cytokines to bias for example the T-cell response like T-helper 1 and T-helper 2, I am not sure whether Dr. Semple would agree that the blood transfusion effect could be mimicked by one or another cytokine. IL-10 is for example a good candidate, because IL-10 is a suppression cytokine. So, concerning early T-cell development, yes I think that there is certainly a need for a good try out of IL-7 in certain clinical settings. IL-10 is already in several trials focused at suppression of immune response.

B. Löwenberg: You are mainly referring to the in vivo application of IL-7. But what about expansion ex vivo, I mean to expand cells and use them for transfusion.

H. Spits: Yes, that is possible although I think that IL-7 alone is certainly not sufficient to expand the pool of T-cell precursors for example. We have done quite a lot of experiments trying to expand precursor cells using IL-7 and indeed you can achieve a limited expansion. But it is certainly not enough for this moment to use that in a clinical setting. Perhaps in the future we will find other factors that can act in concert with IL-7 and indeed develop a method to expand T-cell precursors for clinical purposes.

C.Th. Smit Sibinga: Dr. Touw, I was very much intrigued by the truncation mechanism and the effects truncation eventually has on the remaining molecule. Is this truncation limited to only the G-CSF receptor, or do we see a similar phenomenon in other receptors as well?

I.P. Touw (Rotterdam, NL): Yes, in fact there are now three examples. Truncation of the G-CSF receptor associated with severe congenital neutropenia is the example I discussed; the mutation that was discussed by Dr. Spits in the γ chain of the IL-2, IL-7 and IL-15 receptor is in fact also a truncation mutation, leading to the loss of the docking site – as we call it – for JAK3. The other mutation that I briefly mentioned in the context of benign erythrocytosis is also a truncating mutation. There is also a docking site lost, but this is a docking site for a phosphatase. What is happening there is the phosphatase can no longer inactivate JAK2, which results into an over-activation of the EPO receptor. The intriguing thing is that by roughly the same mechanism, namely truncation of the C terminal domain entirely different functions are being affected. So, JAK3 activation in the SCID system, the unknown maturation signaling properties in the G-CSF receptor and the loss of the docking site for the phosphatase in the EPO receptor.

C.Th. Smit Sibinga: Is the truncation a pure enzymatic cleavage phenomenon or is it based on something different?

I.P. Touw: It is a genetic defect. There is a point mutation in one of the alleles in the haemopoietic cells which leads to the truncation of the protein; so it is a nonsense mutation in the G-CSF-receptor gene that leads to the truncation.

Can I add just one brief comment on the signaling. I briefly touched on the distinct domains and basically the question that you had also relates to this. I think it may be an exciting perspective, if we can modulate specifically the functions of some of the parts of the receptor. I have shown you examples that we can dissect the proliferative signaling from the maturating signaling; this may be a lead to new strategies for, for instance, stem cell expansion. People are now trying to combine cytokines in order to expand stem cells in vitro. An alternative approach might be to use cytokines in combination with substances that interfere with maturation signaling. It could well be that if for example we stimulate proliferation of stem cells with for example IL-6 and at the same time down-regulate the activation of STAT3, that we may be able to expand the cells without letting them go into commitment and maturation. I think this is at least a very exciting area to pursue in models, which may turn out to be interesting for the clinic later on.

H.J.C. de Wit (Leeuwarden, NL): From the presentation of Dr. Semple we learned that the Opelz effect for graft survival is in fact not downregulation of the immune system but is a Th-2 alloimmunisation immune response that gives a better tolerance of grafts. Is there any trick to activate the Th-2 immune response without transfusions, so avoid the transfusion risks and achieve better graft survival, for example the mixture of IL-2 and 8 or a mixture of other drugs to achieve the same effect?

J.W. Semple: Well, in terms of transfusion I do not know any evidence, but in a number of different animal models, for example IL-4 treatment before antigen load can in fact shift the response to a Th-2 like response. So the presence of IL-4 at least in mice appears to be quite important in order to allow those T-cells to differentiate to that type of cytokine production. But in terms of transfusions, I do not know of any evidence to suggest that.

D.C. Dale (Seattle, WA, USA): Dr. Vellenga, I enjoyed your talk about the regulation of cytokine production by monocytes. Do you know how commonly used immunosuppressive drugs like corticosteroids impair cytokine responses particularly at the nuclear level.

E. Vellenga: Corticosteroids I think have different effects. For example when you look at the monocytic cells, one effect is in reducing the production of prostaglandin E2. When you use that, this can also effect the expression of cytokines. Secondly glycocorticoid steroids have an effect on the AP-1 binding sites and there is always a competition between the binding of glycocorticoid steroids and AP-1. So the effect of these drugs is at different levels, prostaglandin, AP-1 and I suppose there should be more signal transduction pathways which are affected by the suppressive agent AP-1.

B. Löwenberg: Dr. Touw, about the impact of the signaling pathways on haemopoiesis. You showed that the importance of the JAK/STAT pathway, which is very directly involved and coupled to a variety of receptor systems. You also showed that there were multiple ways of activating these various STAT molecules. On the other hand the STAT knock outs showed really very little effect in terms of haemopoietic defects. Perhaps it would be useful to hear your explanation for the limited effects on haemopoiesis, particularly in view of your own comment in the discussion that interference and manipulations could perhaps be of practical and clinical use.

I.P. Touw: The answer to your question is basically very simple. Probably the most important STAT molecules for the haemopoietic development may turn out to be STAT3 and STAT5. So, I think it could very well be that STAT3 and STAT5 may be very important for haemopoietic cell development, also in the early stages. Other STATs, e.g. STAT4 and STAT6, have been linked to very specific actions of the cytokines IL-12 and IL-4 respectively. Those are the cytokines that may not have a major role in haematopoietic development, but rather affect immunological responses.

B. Löwenberg: So, one possibility is that the proper STATs still need to be investigated. What about the possibility that we would need multiple knock outs to really get an answer, for instance double knock outs.

I.P. Touw: I am sure that the people involved in this work, which are mostly the groups of Ihle and Darnell in the States, will come up with those double knock outs probably in the near future, if they can survive.

C.Th. Smit Sibinga: Well, there are still a few questions open which I would like to bring forward. There is also information hidden about the efficacy in relation to the half life of cytokines. Cytokines are produced, they are important in the transduction of signals, but do we know about the in vivo half life of the functional capacity of these molecules. What do we know about the degradation of these molecules?

J.W. Semple: Many of these cytokines have very short half lifes. IL-6 for example is in the realm of minutes in terms of biological half life. I think that the host does not want most of these cytokines around, because they tend to cause adverse reactions. So they have evolved mechanisms to get rid of them very quickly.

C.Th. Smit Sibinga: The question is what time span do we then need to have these molecules elicit their efficacy in an in vivo situation.

J.W. Semple: Perhaps the question is, whether or not these molecules are actually causing the responses, or are they indirectly causing the host to secrete cytokines for example; that is not known.

C.Th. Smit Sibinga: You mentioned the phenomenon of these self APCs with the production of allopeptides stimulating the recipient, the auto T helper cell, in the entire alloimmunisation phenomenon. It is known that in a number of situations alloimmunisation and refractoriness disappear in recipients. The question is whether the regular phenomenon through the donor APC and the T helper cells of the recipients is a more durable phenomenon as compared to the phenomenon elicited through these self APCs producing the allopeptide.

J.W. Semple: With the immunosuppressive agents, cyclosporin and FK56, it seems that the direct pathway is less sensitive than the indirect. It possibly is the reason why you would loose HLA-antibodies and therefore refractoriness. On the other hand, it has been shown that immune regulation, such as anti-idiotypic antibodies, may play a role in reducing anti-HLA antibodies.

II. ROLE AND FUNCTION OF CYTOKINES AND GROWTH FACTORS IN THE BLOOD BANK

USE AND APPLICATION OF CYTOKINES AND GROWTH FACTORS IN LABORATORY DIAGNOSTIC PROCEDURES

M. Fujihara, K. Ikebuchi,S. Yamamoto, T. Nakase, S. Sekiguchi

Introduction

Cytokines are potent regulating polypeptides or glycoproteins which mediate a variety of biological and physiological processes involved in cellular and humoral immunity, inflammatory reaction as well as hematopoiesis, and also play important roles in host-defense against infection and tumor growth. Abnormal levels of cytokines and growth factors have been shown to be associated with a variety of diseases. For instance, enhanced IL-1β levels have been reported to be related with sepsis, burn, and rheumatoid arthritis [1-4]. Enhanced erythropoietin (EPO) levels have been found in a series of diseases like certain forms of anemia, and tumors of the kidney or liver [5-7]. Therefore, the information of plasma levels of cytokines as well as growth factors may improve diagnosis, patient follow-up and selection of therapeutic treatments.

Assay of cytokines and growth factors

Bioassay

To measure the levels of cytokines and growth factors, the biological assay and immunoassay are most frequently used. The reverse-transcriptase PCR technique has been introduced to measure mRNA levels of cytokines or growth factors in the limited amount of cells. Table 1 shows bioassays of human cytokines and growth factors. Most of the bioassays are performed by measuring proliferation of factor-dependent cell lines in response to cytokines [8-12]. Some are performed using other biological bases. The chemotactic activity of neutrophils or monocytes is determined for IL-8, MCP-1 and RANTES (*R*egulated upon *A*ctivation, *N*ormal *T* cells *E*xpressed and presumably *S*ecreted) [13-15]. The activity of TNF-α is assayed by cytotoxicity [16], and that of IFN is assayed by induction of viral resistance in EMC infected HeLa cells [17]. Bioassays provide important information. However, bioassay of cytokine level is time-consuming, and may not be specific when applied as a diagnostic marker. Another limitation of bioassay is underestimation of the cytokine activity in sample fluid due to the presence of inhibitors such as soluble cytokine receptors and other antagonistic molecules [18].

Table 1. Bioassay of human cytokine.

Cytokine	Cells	Assay
IL-1	murine helper T cell line, D10.G4.1 human melanoma cell line, A375	proliferation inhibition
IL-2	murine cytotoxic T cell line, CTLL-2	proliferation
IL-3 IL-4 IL-5	factor-dependent human erythroleukemic cell, TF-1	proliferation
IL-6	murine plasmacytoma cell line, T1165.85.2.1 B9 hybridoma	proliferation proliferation
IL-7	PHA activated human PBMC murine C3H/HeJ thymocytes pre B cell line, IxN/2bx (2bx)	proliferation proliferation proliferation
IL-8	human neutrophils	myeloperoixidase release, chemotaxis
IL-9	human megakaryocytic leukemic cell line, MO7e Ts1.C3 cells	proliferation proliferation
IL-10	murine mast cell line, MC/9 IFN-γ synthesis by antigen-stimulated TH1 cells	proliferation inhibition
IL-11	T-1165.85.2.1	proliferation
IL-12	PHA-activated human lymphocytes	proliferation
IL-13	TF-1 B9 hybridoma	proliferation proliferation
IL-15	CTLL-2	proliferation
TNF-α	murine, L929	cytotoxicity
IFN	HeLa cells infected with EMC virus	anti-viral activity
G-CSF	murine myeloblastic cell line, NFS-60	proliferation
GM-CSF	TF-1	proliferation
M-CSF	mouse bone marrow precursor cells	proliferation
LIF	monocytic leukemia, M1	differentiation
CNTF	neuroblastoma, IMR 32	acetylcholine-transferase activity
Oncostatin M	TF-1	proliferation
Gro α/β/γ	cytochalasin B-treated neutrophils	induction of myeloperoxidase
MIP-1α/β	murine hematopoietic stem cell	inhibition
MCP	monocytes	chemotaxis
RANTES	monocytes	chemotaxis
EGF	mouse fibroblast Balb/3T3	proliferation
PDGF	fibroblast line, NR6R-3T3	proliferation
TGF-β	murine IL-4 dependent ^{3}H-thymidine incorporation in HT-2 cells IL-1-dependent thymocyte proliferation	inhibition inhibition

Table 1. Bioassay of human cytokine.

Cytokine	Cells	Assay
Epo	red blood cells of exhypoxic plycythemic mice	incorporation of ^{59}Fe
	TF-1	proliferation
SCF	MO7e	proliferation
FLT3	human myelomonocytic cell, WWF7	proliferation
NGF	TF-1	proliferation

ELISA assay

Recently, monoclonal antibodies against a variety of cytokines as well as growth factors have become available, and using these antibodies, ELISA has been established. Several ELISA kits for the majority of cytokines and growth factors are now commercially available. ELISAs have multiple advantages such as high degree of specificity, ease of performance, and lack of requirements for tissue culture or radioactivity. ELISAs also have disadvantages, including requirements of suitable antibodies or antisera, and detection of proteins such as precursor proteins, denatured or degraded material, and cytokine bound to soluble receptors which have

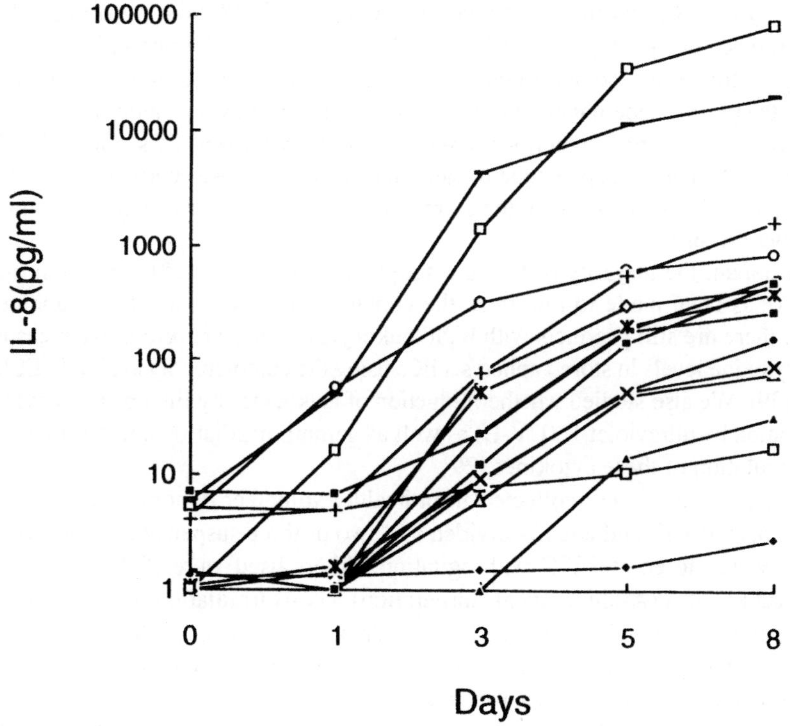

Figure 1. IL-8 levels in stored apheresis PCs. IL-8 levels were measured in apheresis PCs (n=15) sampled sequentially during sotrage. Each line represents the average of duplicate determinations of the IL-8 level.

minimal or no biological activity. In addition, the commercially available kit is still expensive at present.

When different techniques are compared, it is important to consider the presence of interfering molecules in the sample which bind to cytokine, as well as antibodies in the assay system. These endogenous molecules include heterophilic anti-immunoglobulin antibody, cytokine soluble receptor, α2-macroglobulin, complement, and autoantibody. It has been shown that ELISAs are very sensitive to the presence of heterophilic anti-immunoglobulin [19,20]. Complement factors and α2-macroglobulin are also known to be bound to cytokine [21-23]. In addition, the presence of soluble cytokine receptors have been reported in a variety of cytokines [24]. Soluble TNF p55 and p75 inhibit TNF-α biological activity. However, ELISAs can not distinguish free TNF-α from TNF-α bound to soluble receptors.

Application of cytokine measurement in transfusion medicine

Because of the increased availability of the ELISA procedure, many reseachers have measured cytokines in blood components. One of the topics in transfusion medicine is the generation of inflammatory cytokines from contaminating leukocytes during storage of cellular components. A relation to febrile reaction, the duration of storage, and the leukocyte number in PCs was first reported by Muylle et al. [25]. They demonstrated that PCs stored for more than 3 days contained significantly increased amounts of cytokines, including TNF-α, IL-6 and IL-1β. Stack and Snyder [26] reported an increased level of IL-8 in PCs during storage. They also showed that the highest levels of IL-8, in general, were found in PCs with the longest storage period and highest white cell counts. According to Heddle et al. [27], the plasma supernatant, not the cellular component, was mainly linked to the non-hemolytic febrile reactions associated with transfused PCs clinically. The ability of the plasma supernatant to cause febrile reactions was correlated well with the levels of IL-1β and IL-6, the storage period and number of leukocytes in the platelet product.

In Japan, the majority of PCs are supplied by apheresis [28]. Although much effort has been made to minimize the contamination of leukocytes in apheresis PCs, there are still products with high leukocyte counts. Therefore, we measured the cytokine levels in stored apheresis PCs using the commercially available ELISA kits [29]. We also studied whether reduction of leukocytes by filter or leukocyte inactivation by ultraviolet-B (UV-B) as well as gamma-irradiation could prevent the accumulation of these cytokines [29].

Apheresis PCs were collected from healthy volunteer donors by the MCS or Autopheresis CII, and equally divided into two or three suspensions. The suspensions were stored at 22°C with agitation. Filters used were PXL-8 (Pall) and Sepacel PLS-5A (Asahi Medical Corperation). UV-B irradiation of apheresis PCs was performed by Haemonetics Platelet Treatment System at 20,000 J/m^2, and gamma-irradiation by Gammacell 40 at 30 Gy. To detect the cytokine messenger RNA level, standard RT-PCR was used.

Among the cytokines we measured, the production of IL-8 was the most evident. The results of the sequential measurement of IL-8 in 15 apheresis samples are shown in Figure 1. A detectable level of IL-8 was observed at 3 days after storage.

Then, IL-8 levels progressively increased. Two out of 15 apheresis PCs showed more than 1,000 pg/mL after 3 days of storage, and more than 10,000 pg/mL after 5 days of storage. There were good correlations between the initial leukocyte counts and IL-8 levels on day 5 ($r=0.759$, $p<0.05$) and on day 8 ($r=0.719$, $p<0.05$). The question whether IL-8 mRNA production occurred during storage of PCs was tested by the semiquantitative RT-PCR method. Samples without any treatment clearly showed an increase of IL-8 transcripts during storage (Fig. 2). This indicates that IL-8 was indeed synthesized and released from cellular components during storage of PCs.

IL-6, IL-1β and TNF-α showed progressive accumulation during storage of PCs, but the levels of these cytokines were much lower than the levels of IL-8. MCP-I is a member of the chemokine family, like IL-8. The level of this cytokine before storage was relatively higher than those of other cytokines, but there was no significant increase in the level during storage (data not shown).

We studied the effectiveness of filtration, UV-B-irradiation, and gamma-irradiation to prevent cytokine generation. As shown in Table 2, pre-storage filtration was effective. The results of UV-B irradiation and gamma-irradiation are shown in

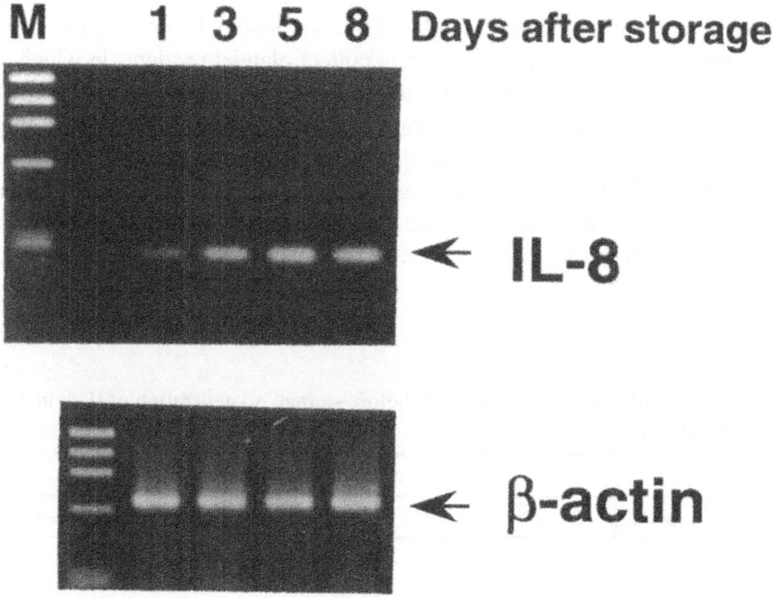

Figure 2. Detection of IL-8 transcripts by RT-PCR. Samples were collected at the time indicated. Total RNA was extracted from the cellular component separated by centrifugation. The design of the primers and the conditions of the PCR reaction have been described previously [53].

Table 2. Effect of pre-storage filtration on generation of IL-8 in 5-day stored apheresis PC.

Unfiltered (pg/mL)	Filtered (pg/mL)
294.5	0.7
625.3	0.8
20.3	0
10.2	5.1
11,755.7	4.3

Table 3. PCs irradiated with 20,000 J/m^2 of UV-B showed a much lower IL-8 level on Day 5 compared with age-matched control PCs, suggesting that UV-B irradiation before storage was effective in preventing cytokine generation. On the other hand, gamma-irradiated PCs generated IL-8 indistinguishable from non-irradiated PCs, suggesting that gamma-irradiation was not effective in preventing cytokine generation.

Consistent reduction of leukocytes in apheresis product by auto-filtration

Figure 3 shows the comparison of residual leukocytes in platelet products collected by various apheresis devices. Platelets collected with current apheresis technology had less than 10^7 leukocytes per bag on average. However, collection with any apheresis device yields some platelet products that exceed acceptable leukocyte contamination levels. Therefore, automatic filtration protocols with Haemonetics MCS 3P were evaluated to collect platelet products in which leukocyte contamination levels are consistently below the acceptable value [30]. We tested two auto-filtration configurations as shown in Figure 4. The in-line filtration employs the filter directly incorporated in the platelet collection line. Platelets were pumped through the filter during surge collection at 200 mL/min. In the on-line filtration, platelets were collected into a temporary bag and then automatically filtered by gravity during the last collection cycle, using two different filters (A,B).

Table 3. Effects of UV-B and irradiation before storage on generation of IL-8 in 5-day stored apheresis PC.

UV-B		γ-ray	
Unirradiated (pg/ml)	Irradiated (pg/mL)	Unirradiated (pg/mL)	Irradiated (pg/ml)
200.0	7.8	1.6	1.9
52.1	7.6	191.5	308.1
191.5	9.2	141.4	97.6
48.9	5.5	14.1	14.1
54.5	23.6	48.9	14.5
556.9	20.3	54.5	174.8

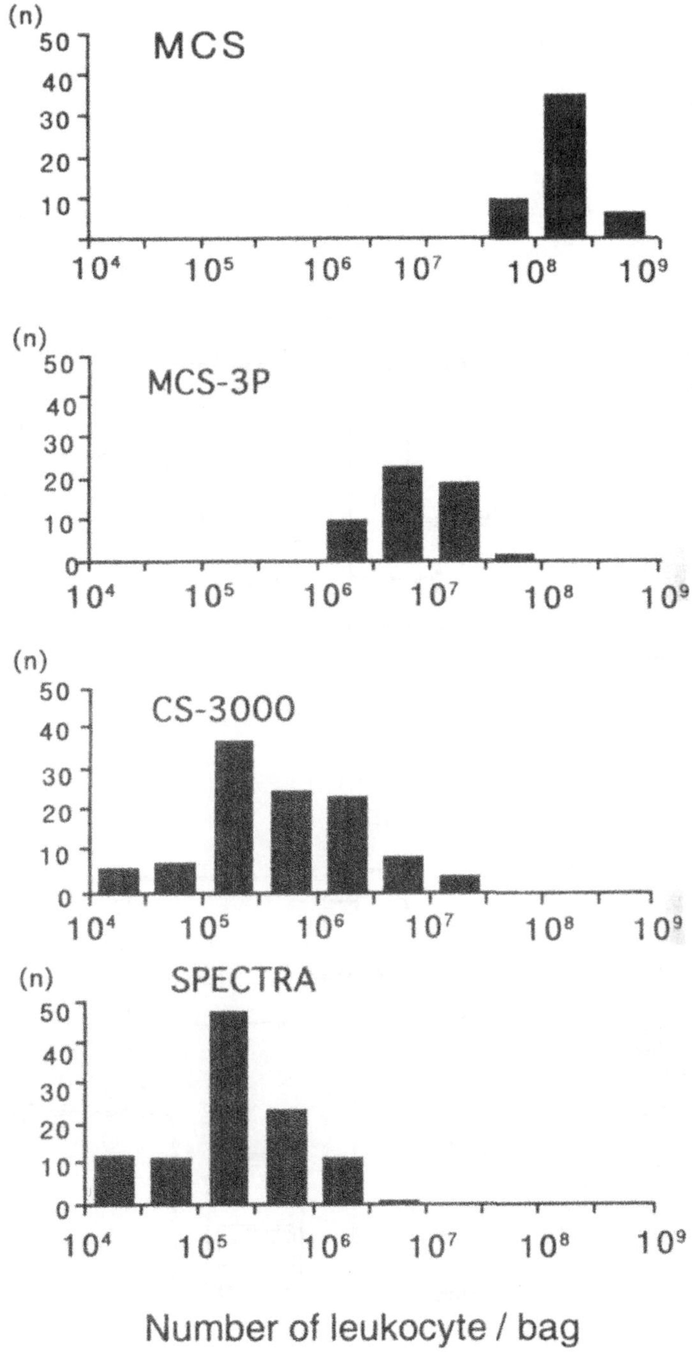

Figure 3. Comparison of residual leukocytes in platelet products collected by apheresis devices.

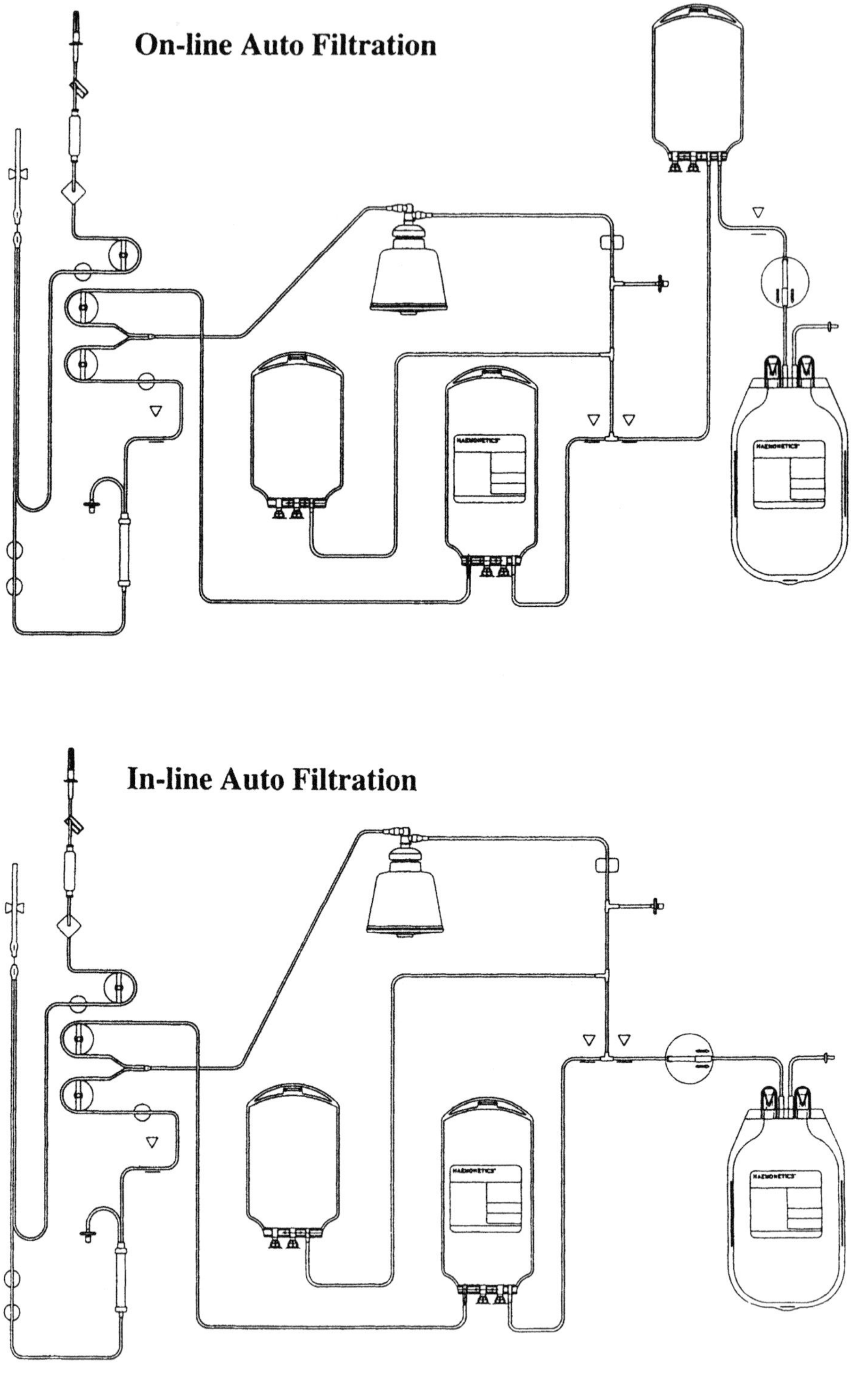

Figure 4. Outlines of in-line and on-line auto-filtration systems.

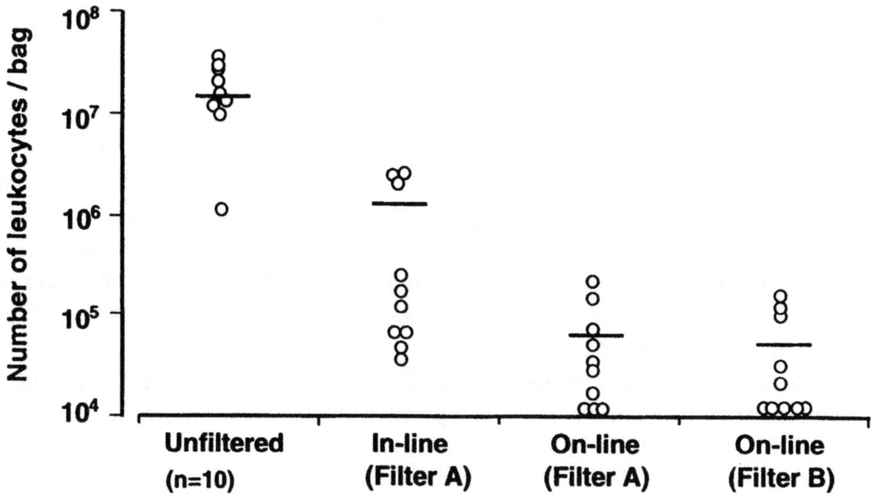

Figure 5. Distribution of leukocyte count in platelet products.

Figure 5 shows the actual distribution of leukocyte contamination for each filtration group. Data from non-filtered platelet collections made on MCS 3P with identical collection settings is also shown. The on-line method of auto-filtration assured a leukocyte contamination level of less than 4×10^5 per bag in all collections. The in-line method resulted in a somewhat higher average leukocyte contamination and greater standard deviation. This was likely the result of the higher filtration flow rate associated with this collection method. Yet, even with the in-line method, all collections had a total leukocyte contamination less than 5×10^6 per bag.

Levels of IL-1β, IL-6, IL-8 and TNF-α were below the detection level over the five-day storage period. In addition, we did not observe any significant difference in the condition or function of the filtered platelets when compared with those of the non-filtered control. Therefore, this new protocol should make a significant contribution toward the routine provision of prestorage leuko-reduced PCs.

Measurement of cytokines generated from platelets in stored PCs

These studies as well as others show that reduction of residual leukocytes definitely prevents the production of inflammatory cytokines from leukocytes in stored PCs. However, recently, Bubel et al. [31] showed that PF4, β-thromboglobulin (β-TG) and RANTES were released from platelets, and accumulated during storage. Wadhwa et al. [32] showed that the production of IL-8 was low in apheresis PCs when compared to platelet-rich plasma (PRP) PCs, while production of TGF-β in apheresis PCs was much higher than that in PRP PCs and buffy-coat PCs. Furthermore, prestorage filtration was not effective in preventing the accumulation of RANTES or TGF-β [33]. RANTES as well as PF4 and β-TG are known to activate basophils, thereby resulting in the release of histamine [34,35]. Therefore, the release and accumulation of such chemokines may be associated with adverse effects such as allergic reactions. This issue should be clarified in the future.

Determination of cytokines in sepsis

The abnormal production of cytokine is closely associated with the etiology of a variety of disorders. Table 4 shows elevated serum cytokine levels in patients with sepsis and multiple organ failure. Increased levels of TNF-α, IL-l, IL-6 and IL-8 have been reported [36-45]. In addition, the peak or sustained levels of TNF-α and IL-6 have been shown to correlate with mortality or severity during infection in several cases, suggesting that the measurement of these cytokine levels in patient serum may be a practical indicator of severity of sepsis [36-40,43,44]. In contrast, Calandra et al. [41,42] reported that TNF-α, IL-lβ and IL-6 were significantly elevated in patients with sepsis compared with non-septic patients, but these cytokines did not give confident cut-off values for the prediction of outcome of individual patients. Therefore, a further clinical study as well as improvement of assay system may be necessary for this issue.

Anti-cytokine strategies have been proposed for treatment of septic shock [46]. Such strategies include reduction of IL-l or TNF-α, infusion of IL-l receptor antagonist, administration of soluble IL-l receptors, infusion of neutralizing antibodies against TNF-α and IL-l, and administration of soluble p55 or p75 TNF receptors. However, clinical trials showed that such anti-cytokine strategies were only effective for patients who had high cytokine levels. Dinarello and Cannon pointed out that one of the values of measuring cytokine in sepsis may be to identify which patients are likely to benefit from anti-cytokine therapy [46].

Determination of cytokines in GvHD and rejection

Elevated levels of TNF-α and soluble IL-2 receptor have been reported in acute GvHD after bone marrow transplantation [47,48]. Miyamoto et al. [48] studied serial changes in the serum soluble IL-2 receptor of patients with and without acute

Table 4. Elevated cytokine level in sepsis and multiple organ failure.

Garaddin et al.	TNF-α, IL-1	Severe infectious purpura	N Engl J Med, 1988
Hack et al.	IL-6	Sepsis	Blood, 1989
Debets et al.	TNF-α	Sepsis	Crit Care Med, 1989
Damas et al.	TNF-α, IL-1	Sepsis	Crit Care Med, 1989
Cannon et al.	TNF-α, IL-1	Sepsis	J Infect Dis, 1990
Calandra et al.	TNF-α, IL-1	Sepsis	J Infect Dis, 1990
Calandra et al.	IL-6	Sepsis	Am J Med, 1991
Damas et al.	IL-6	Sepsis	Am Surg, 1992
Pinsky et al.	TNF-α, IL-6	Sepsis	Chest, 1993
Casey et al.	TNF-α, IL-1, IL-6	Sepsis	Ann Intern Med, 1993
Marty et al.	IL-8	Multiple organ failure	Crit Care Med, 1994

GvHD. They found a significant increase of soluble IL-2R in serum before appearance of clinical symptoms. In addition, the peak concentration of soluble IL-2R correlated well with the severity of acute GvHD. From these data, the authors proposed that the serum soluble IL-2R might be a sensitive and practical indicator for acute GvHD.

During the process of rejection in several organ transplantations, the increased levels of IL-6, TNF-α, soluble IL-2 receptor, IFN-γ, IL-4 and IL-6 have been observed [49-52]. Kutukculer et al. [50] monitored the value of posttransplant IL-2, IL-3, IL-4, IL-6, IL-8, and soluble CD23 in the plasma of renal allograft recipients. They observed that detectable and rising plasma IL-2 levels, whenever they were quantitated, were definitely predictive of graft rejection, and serial monitoring of IL-4 and IL-6 was more reliable for the differential diagnosis of rejection. By contrast, IL-3, IL-8 and soluble CD23 were neither diagnostic nor predictive of rejection.

Further development of the assay technique for cytokines and growth factors will heighten the value of measuring cytokines and growth factors as diagnostic and prognostic markers.

Conclusion

Human cytokine measurements now mostly performed using ELISA procedures and bioassays. Both techniques have advantages and disadvantages. It is important to choose the technique depending on the purpose. The generation of cytokines in stored PC occurs from contaminating leukocytes and platelets themselves. The generation of cytokines from leukocytes in PC can be prevented by pre-storage filtration, inactivation of leukocytes by UV-B irradiation, and preparation of PC with the apheresis device incorporated with in-line or on-line auto-filtration systems. However, the release of chemokines and TGF-β from platelets in stored PC still occurs. The implication of such cytokine release needs to be clarified with regard to the involvement in transfusion-associated side effects.

Plasma cytokine levels correlate with the severity of the disease and the clinical outcome in various diseases (e.g. sepsis, acute GvHD, and acute rejection). The information of plasma levels of cytokines as well as growth factors can be useful as a marker of disease progression or therapeutic efficacy.

References

1. Cannon JG, Tompkins RG, Gelfand JA, et al. Circulating interleukin-1 and tumor necrosis factor in septic shock and experimental endotoxin fever. J Infect Dis 1990;161:79-84.
2. Cannon JG, Friedberg JS, Gelfand JA, et al. Circulating interleukin-1β and tumor necrosis factor-α after burn injury in humans. Crit Care Med 1992;20:1414-19.
3. Eastgate JA, Symons JA, Wood NC, et al. Correlation of plasma interleukin-1 levels with disease activity in rheumatoid arthritis. Lancet 1988;2:706-9.
4. Dinarello CA. Biologic basis for interleukin-1 in disease. Blood 1996;87:2095-147.
5. Jelkmann W. Erythropoietin: structure, control of production, and function. Physiol Review 1992;72:449-89.

6. Hammond D, Winnick S. Paraneoplastic erythrocytosis and ectopic erythropoietins. Ann NY Acad Sci 1974;230:219-27.
7. Kew MC, Fisher JW. Serum erythropoietin concentrations in patients with hepatocellular carcinoma. Cancer 1986;58:2485-88.
8. Gillis S, Ferm MM, Ou W, Smith KA. T cell growth factor: Parameters of production and a quantitative microassay for activity. J Immunol 1978;120:2027-32.
9 Kitamura T, Tange T, Terasawa T, et al. Establishment and characterization of a unique human cell line that proliferates dependently on GM-CSF,IL-3, or erythropoietin. J Cell Physiol 1989;140:323-34.
10. Nordan RP, Pumphrey JG, Rudikoff S. Purification and NH_2-terminal sequence of a plasmacytoma growth factor derived from the murine macrophage cell line P388D1. J Immunol 1987;139:813-17.
11. Aarden LA, de Groot ER, Schaap OL, Lansdorf PM. Production of hybridoma growth factor by human monocytes. Eur J Immunol 1987;17:1411-16.
12. Avanzi GC, Listra P, Giovinazzo B, et at. Selective growth response to IL-3 of a human leukaemic cell line with megakaryoblastic features. Br J Haematol 1988;69:359-66.
13. Schroder J-M, Mrowietz U, Morita E, Christophers E. Purification and partial biochemical characterization of a human monocyte-derived, neutrophil-activating peptide that lacks interleukin 1 activity. J Immunol 1987;139:3474-83.
14. Matsushima K, Larsen CG, duBois GC, Oppenheim JJ. Purification and characterization of a novel monocyte chemotactic and activating factor produced by a human myelomonocytic cell line. J Exp Med 1989; 169:1485-90.
15. Schall TJ, Bacon K, Toy KJ, Goeddel DV. Selective attraction of monocytes and T lymphocytes of the memory phenotype by cytokine RANTES. Nature 1990;347:669-71.
16. Aggarwal BB, Kohr WJ, Hass PE, et al. Human tumor necrosis factor. Production, purification, and characterization. J Biol Chem 1985;260:2345-54.
17. Rubinstein S, Familletti PC, Pestka S. Convenient assay for interferons. J Virol 1981; 37:755-58.
18. Thorpe R, Wadhwa M, Bird CR, Mire-Sluis AR. Detection and measurement of cytokines. Blood Review 1992;6:133-48.
19. Boscaro LM, Stuart MC. Incidence and specificity of interference in two-site immunoassays. Clin Chem 1986;32:1491-95.
20. Boscaro LM, Stuart MC. Heterophilic antibodies: a problem for all immunoassays. Clin Chem 1988;34:27-33.
21. Matsuda T, Hirano T, Nagasawa S, Kishimoto T. Identification of β2-macroglobulin as a carrier protein for IL-6. J Immunol 1989;142:148-52.
22. Borth W, Urbanski A, Prohaska R, Susanj M, Luger TA. Binding of recombinant interleukin-l beta to the third complement and alpha 2-macroglobulin after activation of serum by immune complexes. Blood 1990;75:2388-94.
23. Crookston KP, Webb DJ, Wolf BB, Gonias SL. Classification of α_2-macroglobulin-cytokine interactions based on affinity of noncovalent association in solution under apparent equilibrium conditions. J Biol Chem 1994;269:1533-40.
24. Heaney M, Golde DW. Soluble cytokine receptors. Blood 1996;87:847-57.
25. Muylle L, Joos M, Wouters E, et al. Increased tumor necrosis factor α (TNFα), interleukin-1, and interleukin-6 (IL-6) levels in the plasma of stored platelet concentrates: relationship between TNFα and IL-6 levels and febrile transfusion reactions. Transfusion 1993;33:195-99.
26. Stack G, Snyder EL. Cytokine generation in stored platelet concentrates. Transfusion 1994;34:20-5.
27. Heddle NM, Klama L, Singer J, et al. The role of the plasma from platelet concentrates in transfusion reactions. N Engl J Med 1994;331:625-28.

28. Sekiguchi S. Donor apheresis: recent advances and future development. Vox Sang 1996;70(Suppl 3):126-34.
29. Takahashi TA, Fujihara M, Ogiso C, Hosoda M, Sekiguchi S. Cytokine level determination in stored apheresis platelet concentrates. Transfusion 1995;35(Suppl): 44S.
30. Yamamoto S, Nakase T, Sato N, Ikebuchi K, Sadayoshi S. Automatic pre-storage filtration system for platelet apheresis. Jpn J Med Instrument 1996;66:482-88.
31. Bubel S, Wilhelm D, Entelmann M, Kirchner H, Kluter H. Chemokines in stored platelet concentrates. Transfusion 1996;36:445-49.
32. Wadhwa M, Seghatchian MJ, Lubenko A, et al. Cytokine levels in platelet concentrates: quantitation by bioassays and immunoassays. Br J Haematol 1996;93:225-34.
33. Stack G, Cole S. Accumulation of the cytokines TGF-β1 and RANTES in stored platelet concentrates. Transfusion 1995;35(Suppl):45S.
34. Zuker MB, Katz IR. Platelet factor 4: Production, structure, and physiologic and immunologic action. Proc Soc Exp Biol Med 1991;198:693-702.
35. Bischoff SC, Krieger M, Brunner T, et al. RANTES and related chemokines activate human basophil granulocytes through different G protein-coupled receptors. Eur J Immunol 1993;23:761-67.
36. Giraddin E, Grau GE, Dayer JM, et al. Tumor necrosis factor and interleukin-1 in the serum of children with severe infectious purpura. N Engl J Med 1988;619:397-400.
37. Hack CE, de Groot ER, Felt-Bersma RJF, et al. Increased plasma levels of interleukin-6 in sepsis. Blood 1989;74:1704-10.
38. Debets JMH, Kampmeijer R, van der Linden MPMH, Buurman WA, van der Linden CJ. Plasma tumor necrosis factor and mortality in critically ill septic patients. Crit Care Med 1989;17:489-94.
39. Damas P, Reuter A, Gysen P, et al. Tumor necrosis factor and interleukin-1 serum levels during severe sepsis in humans. Crit Care Med 1989; 17:975-78.
40. Calandra T, Baumgartner J-D, Grau GE, et al. Prognostic value of tumor necrosis factor/cachectin, interleukin-1, interferon-α, and interferon-γ in the serum of patients with septic shock. J Infect Dis 1990;161:982-87.
41. Calandra T, Gerain J, Heumann D, et al. High circulating levels of interleukin-6 in patients with septic shock: evolution during sepsis, prognostic value, and interplay with other cytokines. Am J Med 1991;91:23-9.
42. Damas P, Ledoux D, Nys M, et al. Cytokine serum level during severe sepsis in human IL-6 as a marker of severity. Ann Surg 1991;215:356-62.
43. Pinsky MR, Vincent J-L, Deviere J, et al. Serum cytokine levels in human septic shock. Relation to multiple-system organ failure and mortality. Chest 1993; 103:565-75.
44. Casey LC, Balk RA, Bone RC. Plasma cytokines and endotoxin levels correlate with survival in patients with the sepsis syndrome. Ann Intern Med 1993;119:771-78.
45. Marty C, Misset B, Tamion F, et al. Circulating interleukin-8 concentrations in patients with multiple organ failure of septic and nonseptic origin. Crit Care Med 1994;22: 673-79.
46. Dinarello C, Cannon JG. Cytokine measurements in septic shock. Ann Intern Med 1993;119:853-54.
47. Remberger M, Ringden O, Markling L. TNFα levels are increased during bone marrow transplantation conditioning in patients who develop acute GvHD. Bone Marrow Transplant 1995;15:99-104.
48. Miyamoto T, Akashi k, Hayashi S, et al. Serum concentration of the soluble interleukin-2 receptor for monitoring acute graft-versus-host disease. Bone Marrow Transplant 1996;17:185-90.
49. Kutukculer N, Clark K, Rigg KM, et al. The value of posttransplant monitoring of interleukin (IL)-2, IL-3, IL-4, IL-6, IL-8, and soluble CD23 in the plasma of renal

allograft recipients. Transplantation 1995;59:333-40.

50. Deng MC, Erren M, Kammerling L, et al. The relation of interleukin-6, tumor necrosis factor-α, IL-2, and IL-2 receptor levels to cellular rejection, allograft dysfunction, and clinical events early after cardiac transplantation. Tranplantation 1995;60:1118-24.
51. Kaminski ER, Kaminski A, Bending MR, et al. *In vitro* cytokine profiles and their relevance to rejection following renal transplantation. Transplantation 1995;60:703-6.
52. Umeshita K, Monden M, Tono T, et al. Determination of the presence of interleukin-6 in bile after orthotopic liver transplantation. Its role in the diagnosis of acute rejection. Ann Surg 1996;223:204-11.
53. Carre PC, Mortenson RL, King TE Jr, et al. Increased expression of the interleukin-8 gene by alveolar macrophages in idiopathic pulmonary fibrosis. A potential mechanism for the recruitment and activation of neutrophils in lung fibrosis. J Clin Invest 1991;88: 1802-10.

EX VIVO CYTOKINE PRODUCTION IN BLOOD COMPONENTS: RELEVANT OR IRRELEVANT?

L. Muylle

Introduction

Febrile reactions are frequent complications of the transfusion of blood components. Reaction rates of 6.8% and 37.5% have been reported for red blood cell and platelet transfusion respectively [1]. Whereas the role of leukocyte antibodies, and especially of HLA-antibodies, in causing transfusion reactions was shown in the late 1950's, it was only recently that it became clear that presensitization might not explain the high reaction rate to platelet transfusion [2,3]. Especially the demonstration of an effect of the storage time of random platelets on the incidence and the severity of the reactions and the fact that patients continued to react to platelets – depleted of leukocytes just prior to transfusion – suggested a role of pyrogenic substances accumulated during storage in the plasma portion of platelet concentrates [1,3,4]. These observations led to the examination and the finding of high levels of cytokines, exhibiting *in vivo* pyrogenic activity in stored platelets [5]. Evidence is growing that transfusion of platelet concentrates containing high amounts of these cytokines may cause transfusion reactions [5-7]. The clinical relevance of cytokines in transfusion products will be discussed later in these proceedings by N. Heddle (p. 105).

Besides febrile reactions to transfusion of a high dose of cytokines, there may be other adverse or even beneficial effects. Interleukin-1 (IL-1), interleukin-6 (IL-6) and tumor necrosis factor alpha (TNF-α) belong to a group of cytokines with overlapping biologic properties. They share the ability to stimulate T- and B-lymphocytes, to increase cell proliferation and to promote or suppress the expression of genes for several proteins. They are central mediators of inflammation and the immune response. Special attention will be given to the hematological effects and the question whether such effects may be caused by the dose present in the platelet concentrates.

Generation of cytokines in blood components

The presence of increasing levels of IL-1, IL-6 and TNF-α in the supernatant plasma of random platelet concentrates during storage was demonstrated [5]. Levels of IL-6 increase with more than 3 logs over the base level after 5 days of storage, whereas levels of IL-1α, IL-1β and TNF-α increase with 2 logs after the same storage period. The increased cytokine levels are related to the white blood cells

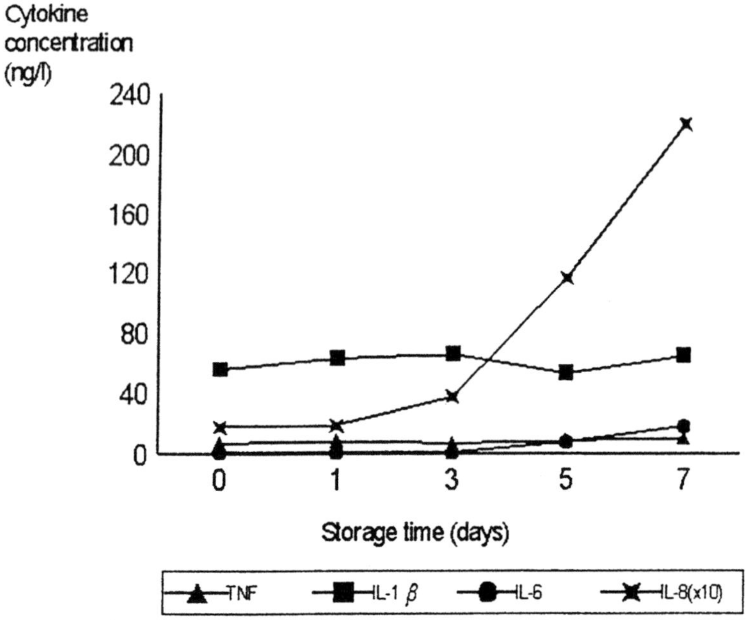

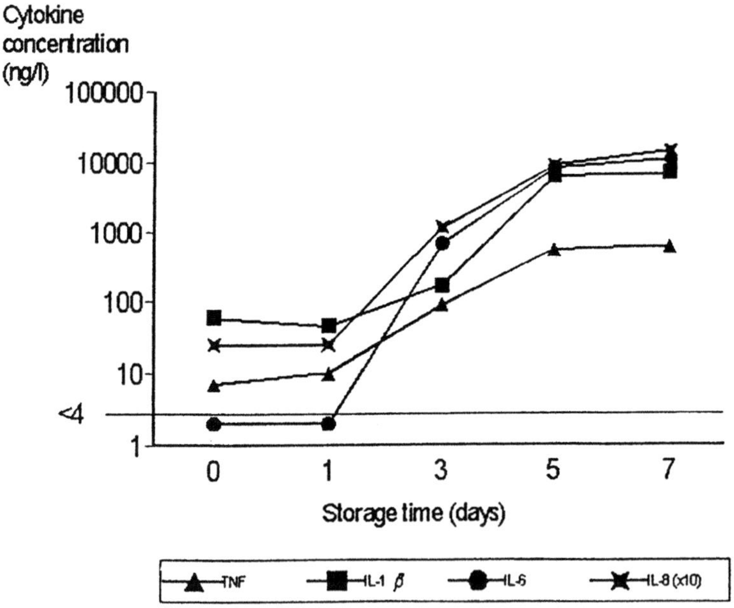

Figure 1. Concentration of cytokines IL-β, IL-6, IL-8 and TNF-α in the plasma portion of stored platelet concentrates (PLC) as a function of the WBC content. A = PLC containing less 3×10^9/l WBC. B = PLC containing more than 6×10^9/l WBC.Data for IL-1β, IL-6 and TNF-α are from ref. 5.

(WBC) present in the container (Figure 1). Detectable IL-6 levels were only occasionally seen in platelet concentrates (PLC) containing less than 6×10^7 WBC per unit. Significant accumulation of interleukin 8 (IL-8) (a neutrophil activating and chemoattractant cytokine) in platelet concentrates was similarly reported by Stack et al., who also showed a direct relationship between WBC counts and the accumulation of IL-8 in stored platelet concentrates. The finding of increased IL-8 in PLC is not unexpected as IL-1 and TNF-α are potent inducers – even at low concentrations – of IL-8 production [8].

The WBC and the plasma of freshly prepared random platelets contain minute amounts of IL-1β and IL-8 and levels of IL-1α and IL-6 below the detection level of the enzyme linked immunosorbent assays (ELISA) [5]. Consequently the increased plasma levels result from an active synthesis and release of the cytokines by activated WBC (monocytes most probably) during storage. Figure 1 also shows that even in the presence of a high WBC count, cytokine levels are not increased after one day of storage. This is probably due to the storage temperature (22 °C) of the PLC that is not ideal for the generation of proteins after activation of the cells. The effect of the temperature on the generation of cytokines is demonstrated by the very small increase of IL-8 and IL-1β during storage of red blood cells at 4 °C, at which temperature cellular metabolism is largely reduced [9].

Because high cytokine levels in PLC are related to the WBC content of the PLC, increased levels are prevented by the prestorage removal of WBC from the PLC using filtration or preparation of the PLC from the buffy coats [8,10-12]. In addition to prestorage WBC reduction, increased cytokine levels can also be prevented by the inactivation of WBC through UV-B irradiation [13]. Gamma irradiation (30 Gy) was found to have little or no effect on the accumulation of cytokines in PLC [13,14].

WBC may be activated to generate cytokines by activated complement components, by thrombin or by cytokines released from WBC damaged or activated by the collection or the preparation of PLC, as it is known that some T-cells respond to subpicomolar concentrations of IL-1 [15]. Once the WBC are triggered, the released cytokines are probably responsible for further WBC activation. However, recent data indicate that WBC may be activated by the non biological surfaces of the plastic container. More adherent mononuclear cells to polyolefin (POF) versus polyvinylchloride (PVC) were found to correlate with higher cytokine levels in POF containers [16]. An effect of the type of plasticizer in PVC – diethylphtalate versus BTHC – was not found (data not shown).

Cytokines in platelet concentrates: amount and factors determining *in vivo* effects

Table 1 gives an idea of the doses of IL-1, IL-6, IL-8 and TNF-α that may be transfused when a pooled platelet concentrate (± 300 ml) consisting of 6 units of random donor platelets prepared by the platelet-rich plasma method is infused into a patient at the end of the five-day storage period. The variety of the cytokine concentrations in the individual random donor platelet concentrates (RDPLC) is very wide. Due to the pooling of RDPLC with high and low content the variation of the cytokine content of the pooled product will be less extreme.

The effects of the transfusion of a stored PLC containing cytokines are – even in the assumption that the doses would be known – very difficult to predict. Reports of the effects of the administration of single (recombinant) cytokines are difficult to compare with the injection of mixtures of cytokines, showing synergism or potentiation, such as found in blood components. Apart from the cytokines measured, PLC may also contain other cytokines and/or substances that influence the effect(s). Furthermore, patient-related factors regulating the cytokine action, such as the degree of receptor expression, the presence of inhibitory receptors, soluble receptors, autoantibodies or receptor antagonists may be important factors in the outcome of an effect.

Table 1. Amount of cytokines infused per transfusion of pooled (n=6) random donor platelets stored for 5 days.

Cytokine	Concentration in RDPLC* mean (range) ng/l	Dose per TRF mean μg	Dose per kg (70 kg patient) mean ng/kg
IL-1β	5,250 (15-26,000)	1.7	24
IL-6	4,880 (<4-17,000)	1.6	23
IL-8	18,000 (470-185,000)	5.9	85
TNF-α	571 (8-1,890)	0.2	3

Data for IL-β, IL-6 and TNF-α: from ref. 5.
* RDPLC = random donor platelet concentrate; TRF = transfusion.

Another problem to be considered when evaluating effects of the infusion of doses of cytokines, that were determined by ELISA's is the lack of standardization of the kits. The lack of standardization of the immunoassays for IL-6 and TNF-α was clearly demonstrated by Bienvenue et al. who showed that depending on the manufacturer the results of the read out versus the National Institute for Biological Standards and Controls (NIBSC) reference standards varied by a factor 30 for IL-6 and 2.5 for TNF-α [17]. To minimize the difference between various commercial sources Ledur et al. recommended the uniform use of the same well-defined international standards for all ELISA kits [18].

Hematological *in vivo* effects of IL-1, IL-6, IL-8 and TNF-α

Morphologically recognizable effects of IL-1, IL-6, IL-8 and TNF-α on the peripheral blood and bone marrow have been reported after the administration of recombinant cytokines in animals and humans.

Ulich reported the induction of a significant neutrophilia accompanied by a lymphopenia 90 minutes after the intravenous (IV) injection of low dose of recombinant human IL-1α and IL-1β (100 U rhIL-1α or β/kg) into rats [19]. The neutrophilia was accompanied by a marked decrease in marrow neutrophils indicating that the source of the neutrophils is at least partly via recruitment of marrow derived neutrophils. At a high dose a rapid neutropenia was noted followed by a neutrophilia 12 hours later. Daily IV injection of low doses IL-1α (0.16 μg rhIL-1α/kg) into rats induced a mild myeloid marrow hyperplasia after 7 days [20]. Effects on the platelet count were not noted. The data of IV or SC IL-1 administration to humans indicate that doses of 2 to 300 ng rhIL-1/kg increase peripheral WBC within several hours [21].

RhIL-6 administered as a single IV injection (0.2-3.2 μg/kg) to rats induced a mild neutrophilia, most likely due to demargination, a mild early lymphocytosis followed by a mild lymphopenia and a reticulocytosis between 12 and 24 hours [22]. Injection of 1.2 μg IL-6/kg caused myeloid and erythroid marrow hyperplasia. Administration of 5 μg rhIL-6 every 12 hours for 5 days to mice produced thrombocytosis after 5 days and an increase in the megakaryocytic size, but no change in the number of megakaryocytes [23]. A dose dependent thrombocytosis was noted after administration of rhIL-6 (0.5-20.0 μg/kg/d) during seven days and a mild leukocytosis during the administration period in patients with cancer before the start of the chemotherapy [24]. A dose related decrease in hemoglobin concentration was also observed within three days of rhIL-6 administration. Given after chemotherapy a faster recovery of platelets occurred without an effect on the platelet nadir [24,25]. A regimen of SC rhIL-6 (30-100 μg/kg/d) administration caused a dilution anemia caused by a rapid increase in the plasma volume [26-28]. In the bone marrow an increase in megakaryocyte size and ploidy without changes in number was reported.

Administration of rhIL-8 (10 μg/kg) to non human primates elicited a rapid and profound neutropenia followed by a rapid neutrophilia [29].

RhTNF in mice and rats (0.5 μg/kg IV) induced an initial neutropenia after 30 minutes followed by a neutrophilia after 2 hours [19,30]. The initial neutropenia may be due to intravascular margination, whereas the neutrophilia is accompanied by a depletion of bone marrow neutrophils suggesting that the marrow neutrophils are the source of the increased peripheral neutrophils. RhTNF-α administered at low doses (2 μg/kg/d IV) for 1 week to rats induced an erythroid marrow hyperplasia and dysplasia of late monoblasts [20]. At high doses (200 μg/kg/d IV) TNF induced a myeloid marrow hyperplasia and an erythroid hypoplasia [31].

Comparison of the cytokine doses found in platelet concentrates (Table 1) with the doses of rh cytokines (reported to cause *in vivo* recognizable effects on the peripheral blood and bone marrow) shows that the latter doses are far above those found in the blood components. Therefore, it is unlikely to expect hematological effects from the cytokines infused along with platelet transfusion. An exception may be an effect of IL-1β on the neutrophil count in the peripheral blood [32].

Recently, a new model of the effector phase of graft-versus-host disease (GvHD) in allogeneic bone marrow transplantation has been proposed [33]. Acute GvHD is seen as a cytokine storm. This storm can be envisaged as a three step process. First, cytokines (IL-1, TNF-α) are released from host tissues as a result of the damage by the conditioning regimen, infection and the underlying disease. The cytokines increase the expression of HLA and leukocyte adhesion molecules on target tissues such as intestinal mucosa, liver and skin. In autologous bone marrow transplantation this process is self-limited and resolves within 7 to 10 days. In allogeneic bone marrow transplantations the first step is followed by donor T cell proliferation when donor T cells, facilitated by their increased expression, recognize the host histocompatibility antigens and become activated. Proliferating donor T cells express IL-2 receptor (IL-2R) and secrete IL-2 and gamma-interferon (IFN-γ) which activate new engrafted mononuclear cells from the donor bone marrow. Finally, the activated donor mononuclear cells secrete additional inflammatory cytokines such as IL-1, TNF-α and IFN-γ, amplifying local organ injury. Endotoxin release by Gram-negative bacteria and production of cytokines such as IL-6 and IL-8 may add to this process.

Large numbers of post-transplant transfusions was one of the variables found to be associated with the risk of GvHD in a multivariate analysis of the data of 2,036 recipients of HLA-identical sibling transplants for leukemia or aplastic anemia [34]. However, it was not clear whether the association respresented a causal relationship or was the effect of existing GvHD. GvHD may affect hematopoietic cells leading to a reduction in hematopoietic cells [35].

TNF-α is a major mediator engaged in early upregulation of GvHD. Holler et al. found a close correlation of maximal systemic TNF-α release (> 100 ng/l) in the first three months after bone marrow transplantation with occurrence of GvHD [36]. They also reported a correlation of increased TNF-α serum levels with the severity of GvHD. The timing of first observation of pathological TNF-α serum levels was even more predictive for development of transplant related complications and overall survival. The highest incidence of complications was found in a group of patients with pathological TNF-α serum levels during pretransplant conditioning. It is very unlikely that the transfusion of a relatively small amount (see table 1) of TNF-α (short half live) could have an effect on the induction or effector phase of GvHD. However it seems wise to avoid – via transfusion of blood components – the injection of extra cytokines in situations with a cytokine dysregulation such as allogeneic bone marrow transplantation.

Conclusion

The presence of high levels of cytokines such as IL-1, IL-6, IL-8 and TNF-α has been demonstrated in stored blood components and can be prevented by prestorage white blood cell removal or irradiation with UVB.

More and more evidence exists that transfusion of platelet concentrates containing high amounts of cytokines may cause febrile transfusion reactions. There is no evidence to expect beneficial hematological effects from the injection of the doses of cytokines as these are found in stored blood components. For the same reason adverse effects on the induction or effector phase of GvHD are very unlikely.

References

1. Heddle NM, Klama LN, Griffith L, Roberts R, Shukia G, Kelton JG. A prospective study to identify the risk factors associated with acute reactions to platelet and red cell transfusions. Transfusion 1993;33:794-97.
2. Chambers LA, Kruskall MS, Pacini DG, Donovan LM. Febrile reactions after platelet transfusion: The effect of single versus multiple donors. Transfusion 1990; 30:219-21.
3. Muylle L, Wouters E, De Bock R, Peetermans ME. Transfusion reactions to platelet concentrates: The effect of the storage time of the concentrate. Transfus Med 1992;2: 289-93.
4. Mangano NM, Chamers LA, Kruskall MS. Limited efficacy of leukopoor platelets for prevention of febrile transfusion reactions. Am J Clin Pathol 1991;95:733-38.
5. Muylle L, Joos M, Wouters E, De Bock R, Peetermans ME. Increased tumor necrosis factor α (TNF-α), interleukin 1, and interleukin 6 (IL-6) levels in plasma of stored platelet concentrates: Relationship between TNF-α and IL-6 levels and febrile transfusion reactions. Transfusion 1993;33:195-99.
6. Heddle NM, Klama L, Singer J et al. The role of the plasma from platelet concentrates in transfusion reactions. N Engl J Med 1994;331:625-28.
7. Muylle L, Wouters E, Peetermans ME. Febrile reactions to platelet transfusion: The effect of increased interleukin 6 levels in concentrates prepared by the platelet-rich plasma method. Transfusion 1996;36:886-90.
8. Stack G, Snyder EL. Cytokine generation in stored platelet concentrates. Transfusion 1994;34:20-25.
9. Stack G, Baril L, Napychank P, Snyder EL. Cytokine generation in stored, white cell-reduced, and bacterially contaminated units of red cells. Transfusion 1995;35:199-203.
10. Muylle L, Peetermans ME. Effect of prestorage leukocyte removal on the cytokine levels in stored platelet concentrate. Vox Sang 1994;66*in vitro*14-17.
11. Flegel WA, Wiesneth M, Stampe D, Koerner K. Low cytokine contamination in buffy coat-derived platelet concentrates without filtration. Transfusion 1995;35:917-20.
12. Aye MT, Palmer DS, Giulivi A, Hashemi S. Effect of filtration of platelet concentrates on the accumulation of cytokine and platelet release factors during storage. Transfusion 1995;35:117-24.
13. Takahashi TA, Fujihara M, Ogiso C, Hosoda M, Sekiguchi S. Cytokine level determination in stored apheresis platelet concentrates. Transfusion 1995;35(Suppl):44.
14. Couban S, Adams C, Klama L, Lee D, Lelton JC, Heddle N. The effect of γ-irradiation on interleukin-1β (IL-1β) and interleukin-6 (IL-6) accumulation during platelet concentrate storage. Blood 1995;86(Suppl):462a.
15. Dinarello CA. Interleukin-1 and interleukin-1 antagonism. Blood 1991;77:1627-52.
16. Davenport RD, Burdick M, Strieter RM, Kunkel SL. Monocyte chemoattractant protein production in red cell incompatibility. Transfusion 1994;34:16-19.
17. Bienvenu J, Coulon L, Doche Chr, Gutowski M-Cl, Grau GE. Analytical performances of commercial ELISA-kits for IL-2, IL-6 and TNF-α. A WHO study. Eur Cytokine Netw 1993;4:447-31.
18. Ledur A, Fitting C, David B, Hamberger Chr, Cavaillon JM. Variable estimates of cytokine levels produced by commercial ELISA kits: Results using international cytokine standards. J Immunol Methods 1995;186:171-79.
19. Ulich TR, del Castillo J, Keys M, Granger GA, Ni RX. Kinetics and mechanisms of recombinant human interleukin-1 and tumor necrosis factor α-induced changes in circulating numbers of neutrophils and lymphocytes. J Immunol 1987; 139:3406-15.
20. Ulich TR, del Castillo J, Guo K, Souza L. The hematologic effects of chronic administration of the monokines tumor necrosis factor, interleukin-1, and granulocyte-colony

stimulating factor on bone marrow and circulation. Am J Pathol 1989;134:149-59.

21. Crown J, Jakubowski A, Gabrilove J. Interleukin-1*in vitro*biological effects in human hematopoiesis. Leukemia and Lymphoma 1993;9:433-40.
22. Ulich TR, del Castillo J, Guo K. *in vivo* hematologic effects of recombinant interleukin-6 on hematopoiesis and circulating numbers of RBCs and WBCs. Blood 1989; 73:106-10.
23. Ishibashi T, Kimura H, Shikama Y, et al. Interleukin-6 is a potent thrombopoietic factor *in vivo* in mice. Blood 1989;74:1241-44.
24. van Gameren MM, Willemse PHB, Mulder NH, et al. Effect of recombinant human interleukin-6 in cancer patients: A phase I-II study. Blood 1994;84:1434-41.
25. Veldhuis GJ, Willemse PHB, Mulder NH, Limburg PC, de Vries EGE. Potential use of recombinant human interleukin-6 in clinical oncology. Leukemia and Lymphoma 1996;20:373-79.
26. D'Hondt V, Humblet Y, Guillaume TH, et al. Thrombopoietic effects and toxicity of interleukin-6 in patients with ovarian cancer before and after chemotherapy: A multicentric placebo-controlled, randomized phase Ib study. Blood 1995;85:2347-53.
27. Nieken J, Mulder NH, Buter J, et al. Recombinant human interleukin-6 induces a rapid and reversible anemia in cancer patients. Blood 1995;86:900-5.
28. Atkins MB, Kappler K, Mier JW, Isaacs RE, Berkman ME. Interleukin-6-associated anemia: Determination of the underlying mechanism. Blood 1995;86:1288-91.
29. Van Zee KJ, Fischer E, Hawes AS, et al. Effects of intravenous IL-8 administration in nonhuman primates. J Immunol 1993;148:1746-53.
30. Remick DG, Kunkel RG, Larrick JW, Kunkel SL. Acute *in vivo* effects of human recombinant tumor necrosis factor. Lab Invest 1987;56:583.
31. Ulich TR, del Castillo J, Yin S. Tumor necrosis factor exerts dose-dependent effects on erythropoiesis and myelopoiesis *in vivo*. Exp Hematol 1990;18:311-15.
32. Trewari A, Buhles WC Jr, Starnes HF Jr. Preliminary report: Effects of interleukin-1 on platelet counts. Lancet 1990;336:712-14.
33. Antin JH, Ferrara JLM. Cytokine dysregulation and acute graft-versus-host disease. Blood 1992;80:2964-68.
34. Gale RP, Bortin MM, van Bekkum DW, et al. Risk factors for acute graft-versus-host disease. Br J Haematol 1987;67:397-406.
35. Chao NJ, Schlegel PG. Prevention and treatment of graft-versus-host disease. Ann N Y Acad Sci 1995;29:130-40.
36. Holler E, Kolb HJ, Hintermeier-Knabe R, et al. Role of tumor necrosis factor alpha in acute graft-versus-host disease and complications following allogeneic bone marrow transplantation. Transplant Proc 1993;25:1234-36.

HAEMATOPOIETIC GROWTH FACTORS FOR THE EXPANSION OF PERIPHERAL BLOOD PROGENITOR CELLS

T.A. Bock, W. Brugger, S. Scheding, B. Ziegler, L. Kanz

Clinical use of peripheral blood progenitor cell (PBPC) transplantation following high-dose chemotherapy is increasingly used in the treatment of solid tumours and haematologic malignancies. As compared with rescue by autologous bone marrow cells, restoration with peripheral blood progenitor cells (PBPC) shortens the period of pancytopenia post transplantation and reduces the risk of infection and bleeding.

A combination of chemotherapy followed by administration of G-CSF or GM-CSF (5µg/kg/d s.c.) usually allows to harvest more than 2×10^6 CD34 positive cells per kg of body weight in most patients. Transplantation of this population after high-dose chemotherapy routinely leads to rapid haematopoietic recovery, mostly with neutrophil counts greater than 500 per cubic millimeter within 10-15 days and platelet counts greater than 20,000 per cubic millimeter within 11-16 days. However, even when extensive numbers of PBPC are harvested and transplanted, further shortening of the pancytopenic period has not been observed.

Unfortunately, there is evidence that PBPC grafts from patients with haematologic or solid tumours are frequently contaminated with tumour cells [1]. Graft-contaminating tumour cells are biologically active and can mediate relapse of neoplastic disease, as shown in clinical retroviral marking studies [2]. Moreover, tumour cells might be co-mobilized together with haematopoietic progenitor cells during chemotherapy and G-CSF-induced mobilization of normal PBPC.

In order to reduce the absolute number of PBPC graft-contaminating tumour cells we positively selected cells carrying the CD34 antigen, using a CellPro immunoaffinity column. Autologous transplantation of these CD34-enriched PC also leads to rapid and complete haematopoietic restoration after high-cose chemotherapy (HDC), and follows an identical time course and pattern as compared to unseparated PB mononuclear cells [3]. By CD34-enrichment, tumour cell load of our grafts can be reduced by 2-3 logs compared to unseparated cells, provided that tumours are not carrying the CD34 antigen and are not enriched, themselves.

In order to further reduce the number of tumour cells reinfused to the patient, *in vitro* culture techniques can be used to expand normal progenitor and stem cells and to provide a biologic purging effect. To harvest only a small number of PBPC and to specifically amplify these cells *ex vivo* to numbers sufficient for transplantation, may then allow to harvest and transplant only a minimum number of tumour cells. For this, conditions are required in which PBPC are expanded *in vitro* – but not contaminating tumour cells. Further advantages include the generation of sufficient numbers of clonogenic progenitors for repetitive clinical use, and to avoid leukapheresis because a small volume of 100ml of PB is sufficient. Potentially, freezing cells would not be necessary since the patients' cells are cultured while the patient is undergoing HDC.

To work out the conditions for this concept, our group has developed an experimental protocol of growing progenitor cells *ex vivo* from a relatively small volume of blood [4]. CD34+ cells were cultured for up to 28 days using mainly RPMI medium, a cocktail of rhCSFs and autologous plasma. All features of the experimental scale protocol had to provide the option for clinical scale application as well. For this reason, a stromal cell layer was not included to feed cultured haematopoietic cells. Numerous conditions and combinations of haematopoietic growth factors (HGF) have been tested in order to obtain optimized yields of colony forming cells. A combination of rh IL-1ß, IL-3, IL-6, SCF, and EPO provided best results in terms of amplification of total mononuclear cells and number of colony-forming cells (CFC) [4], in which the total number of CFC are expanded about 100-200 fold and the maximum of expansion was reached at a two week culture period.

In order to achieve sustained production of mature haematopoietic cells of different lineages after transplantation, it is critical to maintain primitive progenitor and stem cells with extensive proliferative capacity. To test for primitive progenitor cells we assayed long-term culture-inducing cells (LTC-IC) as an indicator for primitive haematopoietic progenitor cells at different time points *in vitro*, and we were able to demonstrate that the number of LTC-IC is maintained for 5-6 weeks [5].

Based on these preclinical data, the ability of *ex vivo* expanded progenitor cells to mediate haematopoietic reconstitution after high-dose therapy was tested in a clinical phase I study [6]. Ten patients with advanced cancer (NSCL, n=5; nasopharyngeal, n=1; breast, n=1; soft-tissue sarcoma, n=1; CUP, n=2) who were eligible for high-dose chemotherapy were included in this phase trial. The patients' age was between 25 and 57 years. Patients received two cycles of induction chemotherapy at an intervall of three weeks, consisting of etoposide (500mg/m^2), ifosfamide (4000mg/m^2), cisplatin (50mg/m^2), and epirubicin (50mg/m^2), a regimen previously shown to be active against a variety of cancers [7]. Twenty-four hours after the second cycle of chemotherapy, the patients received filgrastim (G-CSF; Neupogen, AMGEN) at a dose of 5 microgram per kg of body weight subcutaneously to treat chemotherapy-associated neutropenia and to simultaneously mobilize PBPC. PBPC were collected in a single leukapheresis in which 6 liters of blood was processed [8]. CD34 positive cells were selected by immunoabsorption columns (Ceprate SC; CellPro).

For clinical transplantation, the starting population for *ex vivo* culture consisted of a total of 15×10^6 cells after CD34-selection corresponding to about 10% of the leukapheresis yield. The cells were grown in 2% autologous plasma, rhSCF, rhIL-1ß, rhIL-3, rhIL-6, and rhEpo for 12 days [4]. Non-adherent cells were collected, washed, and resuspended for reinfusion. High-dose chemotherapy (etoposide 1500mg/m^2, ifosfamide 12g/m^2, carboplatin 750mg/m^2, epirubicin150mg/m^2) was administered three weeks after the most recent induction treatment, and expanded progenitor cells were reinfused 24 hours after this therapy. No toxic side effects were observed by infusion of *ex vivo* generated cells [6].

The grafts contained a median of 12×10^6 expanded nucleated cells per kg, representing a 62-fold median increase. Cultured cells gave rise to erythroid, granulocyte-macrophage, and multi-lineage colonies, with a 50-fold increase in clonogenic cells. A median of 1.2×10^5 colony-forming cells (CFC) per kg were generated and transplanted [6]. Four patients simultaneously received uncultured CD34 positive cells in addition to cells generated *ex vivo*, in order not to challenge haematopoietic recovery while possible toxic effects induced by cultured cells were still being evaluated.

Haematopoietic recovery was rapid in 9 patients, while one patient died on day 14 due to neutropenic septicemia. After transplantation of uncultured and expanded cells the median duration of a neutrophil count below 100 cells per cubic millimeter was 5 days (range, 5-7), and median time to platelet counts greater than 20,000 was 12 days (11-15). When expanded cells only were transplanted, neutropenia lasted 6 days (range, 3-11), and thromboytopenia 12 days (11-15). No secondary cytopenic nadir was observed in any patient.

This study demonstrates for the first time the ability of autologous progenitor cells generated *ex vivo* to restore haematopoiesis after high-dose chemotherapy in cancer patients. The degree, time course, and pattern of reconstitution was similar to historical control patients treated with either unseparated mononuclear cells or CD34 selected cells [3]. Since endogenous reconstitution might contribute to long-term haematopoiesis, no definite conclusions can be drawn in respect to long-term capabilities of expanded cells.

To test whether the contaminating tumour cell number had been reduced in expanded grafts compared to uncultured cells and whether tumour cells are co-expanded together with CD34+ haematopoietic PC *in vitro*, cells derived from tumour cell lines were co-cultured with CD34+ fractions at varying ratios [9]. Whereas total MNC were expanded about 100-fold, tumour cells from MCF-7, LXFS, or primary RS-85 were maintained in culture but did not increase in number during two weeks of coculture. Upon replating residual tumour cells into culture conditions that favour growth of these tumour cell lines, tumour cells did regrow and thereby continued to express biological activity *in vitro*. Thus, we have shown that clinical *ex vivo* expansion is clinically feasible and safe, and that normal PBPC are specifically amplified as opposed to tumour cells.

In order to transfer our protocol to complete myeloablative and allogeneic settings, it is critical to clarify whether long-term repopulating stem cells are maintained *ex vivo* using our conditions. Our clinical expansion study could not answer this issue, since endogenous haematopoiesis can substantially contribute to haematopoiesis if HDC is not completely myeloablative, and endogenous haematopoiesis cannot be differentiated or ruled out in an autologous situation. For a long time, there has been no assay for pluripotent haematopoietic stem cells in the human system, since all cells defined and assayed *in vitro* have proven to be primitive progenitors rather than true PHSC, for instance LTC-IC, CAFC, CFU-Blast [10]. As a novel approach, primitive stem cells can be assayed using immunodeficient mice into which human haematopoietic cells can be xenotransplanted and monitored for extended periods [11].

To develop an improved *in vivo* system, we have generated transgenic immunodeficient SCID mice that carry and express the genes for three human growth factors; hIL-3, GM-CSF, and SCF [12]. These transgenic mice support human haematopoiesis for several months, and one can identify and classify these human haematopoietic cells within the murine background. We are currently using this model to pre-clinically test whether *ex vivo* expanded cells do contain human PHSC.

Conclusion

Transplantation of autologous PBPC generated *ex vivo* can restore haematopoiesis after high-dose chemotherapy in cancer patients. No toxic side effects related to the cellular product have been observed. The degree of reconstitution is similar to historical control patients treated with either unseparated mononuclear cells or CD34 selected cells.

A starting fraction of 10×10^6 CD34-selected cells prior to cytokine-induced *ex vivo* expansion yields sufficient numbers of progenitor cells to permit rapid and sustained haematopoietic recovery after high-dose chemotherapy in adults. This number represents about 1/10th of the CD34+ cell number that are used for transplantation of uncultured cells.

Overall, the combined modalities of specific *ex vivo* expansion and CD34-enrichment of PBPC reduces the number of potentially contaminating tumour cells that are reinfused into the patient by 4-5 logs.

Ex vivo expansion appears as an attractive strategy for reducing tumour cell contamination of PBPC grafts. Its future potential includes the generation of sufficient and tumour-cell reduced stem cell grafts, even for repetitive clinical use. Moreover, lineage specific generation of myeloid or megakaryocytic post-progenitor cells might provide the option of further reducing the period of pancytopenia post transplantation. As a prospect, generation of immune cells such as dendritic cells might enable to generate an autologous tumour-specific response starting from CD34+ PBPC grafts.

References

1. Brugger W, Bross KJ, Glatt M, Weber F, Mertelsmann R, Kanz L. Mobilisation of tumor cells and hematopoietic progenitor cells into peripheral blood of patients with solid tumors. Blood 1994;83:636-40.
2. Rill DR, Santana VM, Roberts WM. et al. Direct demonstration that autologous bone marrow transplantation for solid tumors can return a multiplicity of tumorigenic cells. Blood 1994;84:380-83.
3. Brugger W, Henschler R, Heimfeld S, Berenson RJ, Mertelsmann R, Kanz L. Positively selected autologous blood $CD34^+$ cells and unseparated peripheral blood progenitor cells mediate identical hematopoietic engraftment after high-dose VP16, ifosfamide, carbo-

platin and epirubicin. Blood 1994;84:1421-26.

4. Brugger W, Möcklin W, Heimfeld S, Berenson RH, Mertelsmann, Kanz L. *Ex vivo* expansion of enriched peripheral blood CD34$^+$ progenitor cells by stem cell factor interleukin-1β (IL-1β), Il-6, IL-3, interferon-γ and erythropoietin. Blood 1993;81: 2579-84.
5. Henschler R, Brugger W, Luft T, Frey T, Mertelsmann R, Kanz L. Maintenance of transplantation potential *ex vivo* expanded CD34$^+$ selected human peripheral blood progenitor cells. Blood 1994;84:2898-903.
6. Brugger W, Heimfeld S, Berenson RJ, Mertelsmann R, Kanz L. Reconstitution of hematopoiesis after high-dose chemotherapy by autologous progenitor cells generated *ex vivo*. New Engl J Med 1995;333:283-87.
7. Brugger W, Frisch J, Schultz G, Pressler K, Mertelsmann R, Kanz L. Sequential administration of interleukin-3 and granulocyte-macrophage colony stimulating factor following standard-dose combination chemotherapy with etoposide, ifosfamide, and cisplatin. J Clin Oncol 1992;10:1452-59.
8. Brugger W, Birken R, Bertz H, et al. Peripheral blood progenitor cells mobilized by chemotherapy plus granulocyte-colony stimulating factor accelerate both neutrophils and platelet recovery after high-dose VP16, ifosfamide, and cisplatin. Br J Hematol 1993;84:402-07.
9. Vogel W, Behringer D, Scheding S, Kanz L, Brugger W. *Ex vivo* expansion of CD34$^+$ peripheral blood progenitor cells: Implications for the expansion of contaminating epithelial tumor cells. Blood 1996;88:2707-13.
10. Orlic D, Bodine BM. What defines a pluripotent hematopoietic stem cell (PHSC): Will the real PHSC stand Up! Blood 1994;84:3991-94.
11. Dick JE, Lapidot T, Pflumino F. Transplantation of normal leukemic human bone marrow into immune deficient mice: Development of animal models for human hematopoiesis. Immunol Rev 1991;124:25-43.
12. Bock TA, Orlic D, Dunbar CE, Broxmeyer CE, Bodine DM. Improved engraftment of human hematopoietic cells in severe combined immunodeficient (SCID) mice carrying human cytokine transgenes. J Exp Med 1995;182:2037-43.

GENE MARKING AND GENE THERAPY FOR TRANSPLANTATION MEDICINE

D.R. Rill, D. Dilloo, M.E. Grossmann, T. Lemig, M.K. Brenner

The classic application for gene therapy is in the correction of single gene defects, although this has been complicated by the low efficiency of gene transfer into haematopoietic cells. Gene therapy, however, has potential for the modulation of tumour cell growth, drug sensitivity, and antitumour immune responses. In addition, gene marking can be used, in spite of this limited transfer efficiency, to provide information on haematopoiesis, sources of cancer relapse after stem cell transplantation and the relative efficacy of graft manipulation techniques.

Introduction

Although gene transfer is classically associated with correction of single gene defects, little has been achieved thus far in the haematopoietic system because of the efficiency of gene transfer into human haematopoietic stem cells. Whereas single gene defects are rare and difficult to treat many diseases, including cancer, can be attributed to defective interaction among multiple genes. The potential of gene therapy in the stem cell transplantation setting thus extends beyond the correction of monogenic diseases to the modulation of tumour cells growth, drug sensitivity, and immunologic antitumour effector function. These therapeutic applications require gene transfer to be efficient and gene targeting to be precise, often posing considerable difficulty with the clinically approved vector systems. Gene marking studies, in contrast can be informative even with the limited gene transfer efficiency of vectors currently available for clinical trial. In stem cell transplantation, gene marking has been used to answer questions about the biology of normal haematopoietic reconstitution and the effects of cell manipulation on engraftment. Gene marking has also proven instrumental in determining the source of relapse after autologous bone marrow transplantation (BMT) [1-3].

Gene transfer to normal cells

In our initial studies, nucleated bone marrow ($>1.5\times10^8$ cells/kg of body weight) was taken from the posterior iliac crest and two thirds were cryopreserved immediately. The remaining third was separated on a Ficoll gradient to produce a mononuclear cell fraction and was transduced with retroviral vector for 6 hours as previously described [1]. Two retroviral vectors provided by Genetic Therapy Inc. (Gaithersburg, MD) were used for gene marking, first individually and later in combination. Both vectors (LNL6 and G1N) are based on the N2 retroviral backbone and confer neomycin resistance (*neo*ʳ). They are distinguishable by virtue of their different size polymerase chain reaction (PCR) products. At the time of transplantation, both transduced and unmanipulated marrow cells were thawed and reinfused through each patient's central venous line. One month after autologous BMT, the presence of the marker gene in haematopoietic progenitor cells *in vivo* was confirmed by clonogenic assays that showed progenitor marker gene positive by PCR in 15 of 19 patients at one month. The marker gene continued to be detected and expressed for up to 4 years in the mature progeny of marrow precursor cells, including peripheral blood T and B cells and neutrophils. It was also detected in lymphoblastoid cell lines and in cytotoxic T cell lines derived from the patients. The level of transfer varied. In marrow clonogenic haematopoietic progenitors, the average was 5% and the maximum was 29%. In peripheral blood cells, expression was 5-fold to 10-fold lower and was variable between the different lineages. The highest level of expression of seen in myeloid cells, and the lowest level was in B lymphocytes. Delayed appearance of the marker gene in primitive progenitor cells and long-term expression in all three lineages indicated that long-lived multipotent stem cells can be transduced. The levels of gene transfer into haematopoietic progenitors following intensive chemotherapy are higher than predicted from equivalent animal models. This may be attributed to the fact that in our pediatric patient population, the marrow was harvested during regeneration after three cycles of ablative chemotherapy, when a higher than normal proportion of stem cells is in cycle. If it were possible to tranduce haematopoietic progenitors without prior intensive chemotherapy, but with the same efficiency, therapeutic gene transfer approaches might become feasible. Gene marking gives the opportunity to study alternative strategies to induce cell cycling and gene transfer, such as the use of growth factors either given to patients before stem cell harvesting or added to cells after collection. Using a double gene marking protocol as described subsequently for the assessment of different purging techniques, the effects of different combinations of growth factors on engraftment and gene transfer into different haematopoietic subsets can be examined.

Source of relapse after autologous bone marrow transplantation

Although autologous BMT appears to bring about an improvement in survival in many malignant diseases, relapse remains the major cause of treatment failure. The possibility that reinfused malignant cells may contribute to relapse has led to extensive evaluation of techniques for purging marrow to eliminate residual malignant cells. Although it is sufficient to detect the marker gene haematopoietic progenitors to assess normal haematopoietic reconstitution post transplant, it is necessary to identify both the transferred genetic marker and a tumour-specific marker in the same cell population to determine whether residual leukemic or neuroblastoma cells in the autologous marrow contribute to relapse. For example, in one of the acute myeloid leukemia (AML) patients who relapsed, the malignant blasts co-expressed CD34 and CD56, a combination not found on normal haematopoietic cells, and had a complex t(1:8:21) translocation resulting in generation of an AML/ETO fusion transcript that could be identified by PCR. We were able, therefore, to sort blasts expressing CD34 and CD56 and show co-expression in a single clonogenic cell of both a leukemia specific marker (the AML/ETO fusion protein) and the transferred neomycin gene [2]. Four of twelve patients in the AML study have relapsed. In three patients, the malignant cells contained the marker gene, whereas the fourth patient was uninformative, as his blasts did not have a leukemia-specific marker [4]. In the neuroblastoma study, five patients have relapsed, and gene-marked neuroblastoma cells were detected in four of them [3]. In these patients, identification of marked neuroblastoma cells was confirmed by detection of co-expression of the neuroblastoma-specific antigen GD2 together with the transferred marker gene. Four of the neuroblastoma patients relapsed in their marrow, but the fifth had disease recurrence in an extramedullary site in his liver. Biopsy of this extramedullary site showed the presence of gene-marked neuroblast.

Purging studies

We have begun second-generation studies of marrow purging using two gene markers to compare two different purging techniques. In the AML study, one third of the marrow is frozen unpurged as a safety backup. The remaining marrow is split into two aliquots that are marked with G1N or LNL6 and then randomly assigned to purging with initially 4-HC versus interleukin-2 (IL-2) and subsequently 4-HC versus CD15 monoclonal antibody (mAb). At the time of transplantation, both aliquots are reinfused. If the patient should subsequently relapse, detection of either marker will allow us to learn if either of these purging techniques is effective. Fifteen patients have been treated on this protocol as of June 1996, and one patient has relapsed thus far. His relapse was unmarked. Long-term transfer has been seen in normal progenitors, but comparison of the differentiallly marked progenitors from IL-2-purged versus 4-HC-purged marrow fractions indicated that reconstitution of normal progenitors was considerably lower following the IL-2, leading us to abandon this purging strategy.

Neuroblastoma vaccine

Having identified the bone marrow as the source of relapse, we began to use residual malignant cells in bone marrow to generate tumour vaccines. Over the last 5 years, several murine studies have shown that tumour cells genetically modified to express immuno-stimulatory molecules induce an antitumour response not only against the gene-modified cells but also against unmodified parental-type tumour [5]. We chose to assess the tumour vaccine strategy in patients with relapsed neuroblastoma. Several lines of evidence suggest that immune effector functions can influence the course of this disease. Neuroblastoma cells are derived from neuroectodermal tissue that express antigens not present in the normal infant and spontaneous remissions have been observed. Also, sytemic administration of IL-2 has proven efficacious in some patients. We transduced neuroblastoma cells with a G1N-based retroviral vector carrying both the IL-2 and the *neo*^{r} gene. After s.c. injection of IL-2-secreting neuroblastoma cells, a local grade I inflammatory response was observed in all patients. Skin biopsies taken from the injection site demonstrate infiltration of CD8+ lymphocytes 1 week after the injection, resulting in destruction of the injected tumour cells after 2 weeks. Systemic stimulation of the immune system was observed in all patients, with a rise in natural killer (NK) cell-mediated cytotoxicity in most. In three patients, there was also increased killing of the neuroblastoma cell line used for vaccination. In addition, one of these patients developed marked eosinophilia. As levels of IL-2 secreted by the vaccine cells are too low to have any systemic effects on their own, stimulation of systemic immunity is likely attributable to IL-2 in conjunction with tumour antigens presented by the vaccine cells. In two patients, immune activation resulted in regression of tumour. One patient showed regression of pulmonary nodules but subsequently developed progressive disease at other sites and died 8 months later. In the second patients, a lesion of the right humerus regressed by 6 months post vaccination. Biopsies confirmed the differentiation of tumour.

Discussion

Although these initial results with retrovirally transduced neuroblastoma cell lines are encouraging, we aim to improve our neuroblastoma vaccination strategy in two ways. First, the retroviral transduction system has been replaced by an E1, E3-deleted IL-2-adenovirus [6]. This enables us to transduce fresh neuroblastoma cells, avoiding extensive cell culture and possible cell culture related changes in tumour phenotype. We also plan to add a second immunomodulatory component to complement the activity of IL-2 in the vaccine. One candidate molecule that has proven efficacious in our murine leukemia vaccine study is the lymphocyte-specific chemokine lymphotactin [7]. Attraction of lymphocytes to the vaccination site and subsequent expansion with IL-2 afforded greater tumour immunity then was obtained with either agent alone. After completion of the phase I studies with IL-2 alone, we plan to use a similar combination approach for the neuroblastoma vaccines.

Acknowledgements

This work was supported in part by NIH grant CA20180, Cancer Center Support CORE grant CA21765, the American Lebanese Syrian Associated Charities (ALSAC), and the ASISSI Foundation of Memphis.

References

1. Brenner MK, Rill DR, Holladay MS, et al. Gene marking to determine whether autologous marrow infusion restores long-term haemopoiesis in cancer patients. Lancet 1993;342:1134-37.

2. Brenner MK, Rill DR, Moen RC, et al. Gene-marking to trace origin of relapse after autologous bone marrow transplantation. Lancet 1993;341:85-86.
3. Rill DR, Santana VM, Roberts WM, et al. Direct demonstration that autologous bone marrow transplantation for solid tumors can return a multiplicity of tumorigenic cells. Blood 1994;84:380-83.
4. Brenner MK, Cunningham JM, Sorrentino BP, et al. Gene transfer into human hemopoietic progenitor cells. Br Med Bull 1995;51:167-91.
5. Tepper RI, Mule JJ. Experimental and clinical studies of cytokine gene-modified tumor cells. Human Gene Ther 1994;5:153-64.
6. Leimig T, Brenner MK, Ramsey J, et al. Transduction of freshly isolated tumor cells using adenoviral interleukin-2 vectors. Human Gene Ther 1996;7:1233-39.
7. Kelner GS, Kennedy J, Bacon KB, et al. Lymphotactin: A cytokine that represents a new class of chemokine. Science 1994;266:1395-99.

EX VIVO CULTURE AND EXPANSION OF HAEMATOPOIETIC PROGENITOR CELLS IN CANCER PATIENTS

R. Henschler, D. Möbest, F. Rosenthal, R. Mertelsmann

Introduction

Transplantation of the haematopoietic system has become a major instrument in the treatment not only of leukemias in an attempt to eradicate the malignant clone, but also in a number of solid tumours in an effort to increase chemotherapy dose intensity beyond levels of tolerable bone marrow toxicity. Haematopoietic growth factors have been of substantial benefit in improving engraftment kinetics [1]. In recent years, an additional advance has been the isolation of peripheral blood progenitor cells (PBPC) as a source of transplantable haematopoietic stem cells. PBPC have been shown to mediate earlier platelet and neutrophil recovery compared to bone marrow [2-5] A range of studies is under way investigating clinical benefit for patients transplanted with PBPC in a variety of disease states, including Non-Hodgkin's lymphomas, Hodgkin's disease, acute leukemias as well as some chemosensitive solid tumours [6 for review].

Since it has been recognized that bone marrow or PBPC might still contain tumour cells in a proportion of patients with certain solid tumours as well as lymphomas [7-9] purging strategies have been designed to obtain tumour clean transplants. One first step to deplete PBPC samples of tumour cells is to enrich for CD34 positive cells, since the marrow repopulating stem cells reside in the CD34+ compartment [10]. The development of high affinity CD34 antibodies has led to the design of immunoaffinity systems that have now entered clinical trials [e.q. 11].

Before devices to enrich for primitive haematopoietic cell populations on a large scale had been at hand, the *ex vivo*, i.e. *in vitro* growth of cell fractions derived from bone marrow had been notoriously difficult. The main reasons for this may have been the relatively low stem cell content of unseparated mononuclear cell populations, and the ability of mature cells present in these populations to produce a number of cytokines negatively interfering with progenitor growth. Clinical grade CD34+ selection generating highly enriched CD34+ populations has been a major step forward to improve subsequent *ex vivo* expansion of haematopoietic cells in liquid culture. Another difficulty was, that a smaller number of polypeptide growth factors had been available at the time as recombinant material that could be used to drive haematopoietic cell proliferation in culture. The advent of Stem Cell Factor (SCF) initiated a major change of this situation in 1990 [12].

Rationale for *ex vivo* expansion of PBPC

One rationale for *ex vivo* expansion of haematopoietic cells is to provide amplified numbers of progenitor cells in a transplant, assuming that committed progenitors are mediators of early PBPC engraftment. This may be of importance to further shorten neutropenic and thrombocytopenic periods in patients during postchemotherapy aplasia. The principle of progenitor amplification may also be of benefit when stem cell yields in PBPC or bone marrow harvests are too low for a conventional transplant and sufficient numbers of progenitor cells can be generated by *ex vivo* expansion. On the other hand, *ex vivo* expansion may start from a relatively small amount of whole blood as starting material (500 ml or less), thus obviating the need for leukapheresis or bone marrow harvest procedures.

Another major goal of *ex vivo* expansion is its possible use as a tool for tumour cell purging by creating growth conditions adverse for malignant cells but spurring haematopoietic cell survival, expansion and development. Lastly, successful *ex vivo* culture of PBPC is the prerequisite for gene transfer into the haematopoietic system. These points are listed in Table 1.

Table 1. Rationale for *ex vivo* expansion of haematopoietic progenitor cells.

- Amplify numbers of colony forming cells to enforce engraftment
- Amplify intermediate stages of hematopoietic differentiation underrepresented in PBSC autografts
- Generate sufficient numbers of CFC from patients with low PBPC yields
- Avoid leukapheresis or bone marrow harvest under general anesthesia
- Deplete of tumour cells contaminating the PBPC preparation
- Provide environment to genetically manipulate hematopoitic stem and progenitor cells

Protocols for *ex vivo* expansion cultures

It has been demonstrated that human bone marrow, peripheral blood or cord blood stem cells may be cultured in the absence of stroma cells, provided that a minimum amount and number of growth factors and, in most cases, serum is present. Moore and coworkers have described a stroma free continuous culture system, growing progenitor cells over periods of several weeks, that can be used to assay for the progenitor content of stem cell grafts ["Delta Assay", 13]. Depending on the quality and quantity of growth factors added, different plateau levels in the maximum achieved number of colony forming cells (CFC) generated in these cultures from a given stem cell population. These cultures reflected to a high degree the different proliferation capacities of early, uncommitted or partially committed progenitors in response to colony stimulating factors (CSF). For example, SCF is mainly acting as a survival factor, when alone, or increasing proliferation and differentiation of stem cells in synergy with other CSFs; interleukin-1 beta (IL-1β) is mainly acting on progenitors with high proliferative capacity [13]. These studies formed the methodological basis to further develop stroma free culture system for use in therapy.

When the mononuclear fraction from PBPC harvests is cultured in the presence of SCF and PIXY 321, a GM-CSF/IL-3 fusion protein, CFU-GM colony forming cells could be expanded by a factor of more than 15 within 8 days [14]. These cultures contained fetal calf serum. At the same time, an expansion of erythroid colonies (BFU E) by a factor of 10 was achieved. Haylock et al. [15] used purified CD34+ PBPC cells as starting material and a combination of up to six haematopoietic growth factors. They readily obtained a more than 2 log amplification of total cell numbers over a 2 week culture period, consisting predominantly of immature neutrophil like cells; no expansion of CFC was noted. These authors focused their approach primarily on the generation of neutrophil precursors of a maturation state more terminal than the colony forming cell, as this maturational state of precursors is not normally present in substantial numbers in peripheral blood progenitor harvests and may thus be able to confer production of mature neutrophils within a shorter interval post transplantation than seen with PBPC. Teofili et al. [16] saw that PBPC CD34+ cells yielded higher expansion of cell numbers than bone marrow derived CD34+ cells, using a combination of five growth factors, SCF, GM-CSF, IL-1, IL 3 and IL-6. They noted increases in colony forming cell numbers after seven days of culture, whereas CFC numbers declined in the second week of culture. In a liquid culture system of PBPC CD34+ cells established at our institution, amplification of CFC by a factor of up to 190 fold was measured after two weeks of culture in a combination of five growth factors, SCF, IL-1, IL-3, IL-6 and erythropoietin (EPO) in the presence of fetal calf serum [17]. In this system, the main emphasis was to amplify the number of colony forming cells, since a number of studies transplanting PBPC had described inverse correlations between the number of CFC reinfused into patients and the period of absolute neutropenia [e.g., 18].

Starting cell populations

From the studies mentioned above, it became clear that cultures derived from CD34+ cells showed a much more sustained cell proliferation of up to six weeks in culture than cultures initiated with unseparated mononuclear cell fractions, provided the cultures were refed and cells diluted at, in most cases, weekly intervals.

Attempts have been made to identify highly enriched populations of primitive progenitor cells by more extensive enrichment techniques such as flow cytometric cell sorting. For example, CD34+, HLA DR-, CD15- Rhodamin^{dull} cell populations separated by flow cytometry were able to further enhance the maximum increase in cell numbers in expansion cultures to more than 1,500 fold, expanding at the same time different types of progenitor cells including high proliferative potential-CFC [19]. Among three different sorted stem cell population from human umbilical cord blood, one was found to contain predominantly multipotent progenitors (CD34+ CD45RA^{low} CD71^{low}), one to contain predominantly myeloid progenitors (CD34+ CD45RA+ CD71^{low}), and one to contain predominantly erythroid progenitors (CD34+ CD45RA^{low} CD71+). The population containing most of the multipotent precursors (CD34+ CD45RA^{low} CD71^{low}) showed the highest expansion rate of CD34+ cell numbers after two weeks of culture in a growth factor supplemented serum free medium (532 fold versus 130 and 28 fold, respectively [20]. Another surface molecule useful to further enrich for primitive cells from this cell population is the Thy-1 antigen [21].

During their ontogeny, haematopoietic stem cells display a decrease in their *in vitro* proliferative potential [22] This makes cord blood stem cells a potentially very attractive starting cell population for *ex vivo* expansion. However, for therapeutic use of expanded cells in autologous transplantation, PBPC (or bone marrow) may be the source of highest relevance because cord blood is usually not available for these patients.

Therapeutic application of *ex vivo* expanded cells

At our institution, *ex vivo* expanded CD34+ PBPC were reinfused into patients undergoing dose escalated chemotherapy in a phase I study [23]. 1/10 of a single 2 hour leukapheresis product was expanded for two weeks in the presence of CSF, IL-1, IL-3, IL-6, EPO, and autologous serum. The reconstitution pattern in the patients receiving more than 1×10^5 CFU-GM/kg was identical to historical patients receiving CD34+ selected or unselected PBPC (Table 2). Periods of absolute neutropenia and thrombopenia were between 4 and 7 days and thus were significantly (approximately one week) shorter than in historical controls reveiving no stem cell support, but identical high dose chemotherapy and growth factor support post chemotherapy (Table 2). This indicates that *ex vivo* expanded cells may be useful to confer (at least) short term engraftment after the above mentioned high dose chemotherapy protocol which normally results in an aplasia period of approximately three weeks without progenitor cell reinfusion and growth factor application.

It is not known, however, to which degree *ex vivo* expanded blood stem cells may result in long term engraftment, which will be needed after total body irradiation and/or myeloablative high dose chemotherapy. These experiments have not been performed in man yet. Muench et al. [24] transplanted mice with enriched bone marrow stem cells expanded *ex vivo* by IL-1, IL-6 and SCF. They demonstrated long term donor-derived haematopoiesis in the transplanted animals. Similarly, Rebel et al. [25] have observed maintenance and amplification of primitive haematopoietic stem cells defined by the surface markers, Sca-1+ and wheat germ agglutinin+, that were negative for lineage markers, in a serum free culture system from murine bone marrow, starting from an enriched population of stem cells.

Long term bone marrow culture is considered the most useful biological *in vitro* assay available measuring cells potentially capable of long term haematopoietic reconstitution [26]. In our *ex vivo* expanded CD34+ PBPC, we have analysed the

Table 2. Recovery times using PBPC and *ex vivo* expanded cells post high dose chemotherapy with VP-16, ifosfamide, and cisplatin in patients with solid tumours.

Source of transplant	**CSFs post chemotherapy**	**Neutrophils <100/µl (days)**	**Platelets <20.000/µl (days)**	**No. of patients**
–	G-CSF	10.5	8	6[1)]
PBPC	G-CSF	6.5	3	8[1)]
Ex vivo expanded CD34+ PBPC	G-CSF	7	4	3[2)]

Data from [5, 23]. All values represent median values.

1. Patients received high dose chemotherapy with VP-16 (1500 mg/m^2), ifosfamide (12 g/m^2), and cisplatin (150 mg/m^2).
2. Patients received high dose chemotherapy with VP-16 (1500 mg/m^2), ifosfamide (12 g/m^2), carboplatin (750 mg/m^2) and epirubicin (150 mg/m^2).

content of "Long Term Bone Marrow Culture initiating cells" [LTCIC, 27]. Overall, LTCIC could not be amplified during *ex vivo* expansion. They could, however, be maintained approximately at input levels if SCF, IL-l, IL-3, IL-6 and EPO were all present during the expansion culture. A different method, fluorescent dye tracking, identified a fraction of primitive human bone marrow stem cells that were not recruited into cell division by a combination of IL-3, IL-6 and SCF and EPO in culture [28]. At the same time, *ex vivo* expansion took place in these cultures from more committed progenitor cells. Verfaillie et al. [29] identified a culture medium composed of IL-3, Macrophage Inflammatory Protein 1 alpha and unknown activities secreted from stromal cells, that was able to maintain LTCIC in culture for at least eight weeks.

Systematic improvement of culture conditions in bioreactor systems

Besides the exploration of the capability of recombinant haematopoietic growth factors combinations to optimally support growth and development in *ex vivo* expansion cultures, more and more attention is now being paid to technical improvements of culture conditions. This includes the effects of continuous medium flow, rapid medium exchange, ion, lipid and protein content in the cultures, oxygen tension and other components in the liquid phase of the culture system, as well as growth of progenitor cells on specially designed surface structures.

We observed concentration-dependent inhibition of expansion rates by the addition of autologous patient serum in a number of samples. In our hands, use of serum free medium resulted in, compared to serum-containing cultures, more reliable and overall enhanced cell production of up to 400 fold within 12 days. A forced medium exchange (50% medium change every day), resulted in a 2.5 fold better amplification rates in a system used by Schwartz [30]. This correlated with an increased glucose consumption in these cultures [31]. A more recent publication noted that the presence of a stroma layer and increased feeding schedules had a greater beneficial effect on amplification or survival of CFU-GM and LTCIC than alterations of cytokine concentrations and cytokine combinations used [32].

A logical next step from the results with enhanced feeding protocols was the use of perfused culture systems. The most simple improvement here investigated by Zandstra et al. [33] achieved substantially higher cell yields as compared to static cultures by just adding a continuously rotating stirrer to their culture bottle. In a system used by Koller et al. [34] it was noted that the depletion of glucose and IL-3, as well as the accumulation of lactate and IL-6 observed in static cultures could be circumvented in continuously perfused cultures. These authors also found that an oxygen content of 5% was superior to the normal oxygen content of 20% to achieve maximum progenitor and total cell expansion [35]. Moreover, continuous perfusion cultures seemed to allow an expansion also of LTCIC.

The cellular microenvironment has been another focus of research in this field. Oh et al. [36] saw extended growth when newly produced cells were harvested periodically from the bioreactor, and assumed that enhancement of the available growth surface was responsible for this effect. A three-dimensional artificial microenvironment was introduced by Naughton et al. [37] using suspended nylon screens, that could sustain bone marrow cultivation for 270 days in model using rat marrow cells, and for 12 weeks using human bone marrow cells. Its usefulness for *ex vivo* expansion has not been analyzed yet, however. Davis et al. [38] described a hollow fibre system consisting of porcine microvascular endothelial cells, improving *ex vivo* expansion of human bone marrow CD34+ cells. Similarly, the use of two chambers separating the haematopoietic cells from continuously flowing medium by dialysis membranes, created a microenvironment allowing continuous proliferation and maturation of, in this case, murine bone marrow cells [39]. Again, this system has not been tested for *ex vivo* expansion. One may speculate that in future, these aspects of culture technique will gain increasing importance. Another trend will probably be the development of more handy, technically easy and uncomplicated systems, uniting the most important characteristics of the bioreactors mentioned above.

References

1. Lieschke G. Burgess AW. Granulocyte colony-stimulating factor and granulocyte-macrophage colony-stimulating factor. N Engl J Med 1992;327:28-35,99-106.
2. Sheridan WP, Begley CG, Juttner CA, et al. Effect of peripheral blood progenitor cells mobilized by filgrastim (G-CSF) on platelet recovery after high dose chemotherapy. Lancet 1992;339:640-44.
3. Elias AD, Ayash L, Anderson KC, et al. Mobilization of peripheral blood progenitor cells by chemotherapy and granulocyte-macrophage colony-stimulating factor for hematologic support after high dose intensification in breast cancer. Blood 1992;79:3036-44.
4. To LB, Roberts MM, Haylock DN, et al. Comparison of hematological recovery times and supportive care requirements of autologous recovery phase peripheral stem cell transplants, autologous bone marrow transplants and allogeneic bone marrow transplants. Bone Marrow Transplant 1992;9:277-84.
5. Brugger W, Birken R, Bertz H, H et al. Peripheral blood progenitor cells mobilized by chemotherapy + G-CSF accelerate both neutrophil and platelet recovery after high dose VP16, ifosfamide and cisplatin. Br J Haematol 1993;84:402-07.

6. Kessinger A, Armitage JO. The evolving role of autologous peripheral stem cell transplantation following high dose chemotherapy for malignancies. Blood 1991;77:211-13.
7. Ross AA, Cooper BW, Lazarus HM, et al. Detection and viability of tumour cells in peripheral blood stem cell collections from breast cancer patients using immunocytochemical and clonogenic assay techniques. Blood 82.1993;82:2605-10.
8. Sharp JG, Bishop M, Chan WC et al. Detection of minimal residual disease in hematopoietic tissues. Ann N Y Acad Med 1995;770:242-6l.
9. Brugger w, Bross KJ, Glatt M, Weber F, Mertelsmann R, Kanz L. Mobilization of tumour cells and hematopoietic progenitor cells into peripheral blood of patients with solid tumours. Blood 1994;83:636-40.
10. Berenson RJ, Andrews RG, Bensinger WI, et al. Antigen CD34+ marrow cells engraft lethally irradiated baboons. J Clin Invest 1988;81:951-55.
11. Berenson RJ, Bensinger WI, Hill RS, et al. Engraftment after infusion of CD34+ marrow cells in patients with breast cancer or neuroblastoma. Blood 1991;77:1717-22.
12. Witte ON. Steel locus defines new multipotent growth factor. Cell 1990;63:5-6.
13. Moore MA. Clinical implications of positive and negative stem cell regulators. Blood 1991; 78:1-19.
14. McAlister IB, Teepe M, Gillis S, Williams DE. *Ex vivo* expansion of peripheral blood progenitor cells with recombinant cytokines. Exp Hematol 1992;20:626-28.
15. Haylock DN, To LB, Dowse TL, Juttner CA, Simmons PJ. *Ex vivo* expansion and maturation of peripheral blood CD34+ cells into the myeloid lineage. Blood 1992;80: 1405-12.
16. Teofili L., Iovino M, Di Mario A, et al. *In vitro* expansion of CD34+ cells mobilized with chemotherapy and G-CSF. Int J Artif Organs 1993;16(Suppl 5):89-95.
17. Brugger W, Möcklin W, Heimfeld S, Berenson RJ, Mertelsmann R, Kanz L. *Ex vivo* expansion of enriched peripheral blood CD34+ progenitor cells by stem cell factor, interleukin-1β, IL-6, IL-3, interferon-gamma, and erythropoietin. Blood 1993;81: 2579-84.
18. Pettengell R, Testa NG, Swindell R. Crowther D, Dexter TM. Transplantation potential of hematopoietic cells released into the circulation during routine chemotherapy for Non-Hodgkin's Lymphoma. Blood 1993;82:2239-48.
19. Srour EF, Brandt JE, Bridell RA , Gringsby S, Leemhuis T, Hoffman R. Long term generation and expansion of human primitive hematopoietic progenitor cells *in vitro*. Blood 1993;81:661-69.
20. Mayani H, Dragowska W, Lansdorp PM. Lineage commitment in human hemopoiesis involves asymmetric cell division of multipotent progenitors and does not appear to be influenced by cytokines. J Cell Physiol 1993;157:579-86.
21. Mayani H, Dragowska W, Lansdorp PM. Characterization of functionally distinct subpopulations of CD34+ cord blood cells in serum-free long term cultures supplemented with hematopoietic cytokines. Blood 1993;82:2664-72.
22. Lansdorp P M, Dragowska W, Mayani H. Ontogeny related changes in proliferative potential of human hematopoietic cells. J Exp Med 1993;178:787-91.
23. Brugger W, Heimfeld S, Berenson RJ, Färber L, Mertelsmann R, Kanz L. Reconstitution of hematopoiesis after high dose chemotherapy by autologous progenitor cells expanded *ex vivo*. N Engl J Med 1995;333:283-87.
24. Muench MO, Firpo MT, Moore MAS. Bone marrow transplantation with interleukin-1 plus kit-ligand *ex vivo* expanded bone marrow accelerates hematopoietic reconstitution in mice without loss of stem cell lineage and proliferative potential. Blood 1993;81: 3463-73.
25. Rebel VI, Dragowska W, Eaves CJ, Humphries RK, Lansdorp PM. Amplification of Sca-1+ Lin−WGA+ cells in serum free cultures containing steel factor, interleukin-6,

and erythropoietin with maintenance of cells with long-term *in vivo* reconstituting potential. Blood 1994;83:128-36.
26. Testa NG, Dexter TM. The biology of long-term bone marrow cultures and its application to bone marrow transplantation. Curr Opin Oncol 1992;3:272-78.
27. Henschler R, Brugger W, Luft T, Frey T, Mertelsmann R, Kanz L. Maintenance of transplantation potential in *ex vivo* expanded human CD34+ peripheral blood progenitor cells. Blood 1994;84:2898-903.
28. Lansdorp P M, Dragowska W. Maintenance of hematopoiesis in serum free bone marrow cultures involves sequential recruitment of quiescent progenitors. Exp Hematol 1993;21:1321-27.
29. Verfaillie CM, Catanzarro PM, Li WN. Macrophage inflammatory protein 1-alpha, interleukin-3, diffusible marrow stroma factors maintain human hematopoietic stem cells for at least eight weeks *in vitro*. J Exp Med 1994;179:643-49.
30. Schwartz RM, Palsson BO, Emerson SG. Rapid medium perfusion rate significantly increases the productivity and longlivity of human bone marrow cultures. Proc Natl Acad Sci USA 1991;88(15):6760- 64.
31. Caldwell J, Palsson BO, Locey B, Emerson SG. Culture perfusion schedules influence the metabolic activity and granulocyte macrophage colony- stimulating factor production rates of human bone marrow stromal cells. J Cell Physiol 1991;147:344-53.
32. Koller MR, Palsson MA, Manchel I, Newsom BS, Van Zant G, Palsson BO. Expansion of CD34-enriched human bone marrow cells: Effect of feeding schedule, cytokines, and stroma. Exp Hematol 1994;22:726.
33. Zandstra PW, Cameron G, Eaves CJ, Pieret JM. Hematopoietic progenitor cell expansion in stirred suspension reactors. Blood 1994;84(Suppl 1):498a.
34. Koller MR, Palsson MA, Manchel I, Palsson BO. Long-term culture initiating cell expansion is dependent on frequent medium exchange combined with stromal and other accessory cell effects. Blood 1995;86:1784-93.
35. Koller MR, Bender JG, Papoutsakis ET, Miller WM. Beneficial effects of reduced oxygen tension and perfusion in long-term hematopoietic cultures. Ann N Y Acad Sci 1992;665:105-16.
36. Oh DJ, Koller MR, Palsson BO. Frequent harvesting from perfused bone marrow cultures results in increased overall cell and progenitor expansion. Biotechnol Bioeng 1994;4:609-16.
37. Naughton BA, Tjota A, Sibanda B, Naughton GK. Hematopoiesis on suspended nylon screen-stromal cell microenvironments. J Biomech Eng 1991;113:171-77.
38. Sardoni CA, Wu YJ. Expansion and differentiation of human hematopoietic cells from static cultures through small-scale bioreactors. Biotech Prog 1993;9:131-37.
39. Wang T-Y, Brennan JK, Wu JHD. Multilineal hematopoiesis in a three-dimensional murine long-term bone marrow culture. Exp Hematol 1995;22:26-32.

PERIPHERAL BLOOD PROGENITOR GRAFTS OBTAINED FROM HEALTHY DONORS

P. Dreger, N. Schmitz

Introduction

After the first cases of allogeneic transplantation of G-CSF-primed peripheral blood prognitor cells (PBPC) had been reported a few years ago [1,2] the use of mobilized PBPC instead of BM as source of allogeneic stem cells has rapidly expanded [3]. The present article will elucidate the potential benefits and limitations of allogeneic PBPC with particular focus on collection and cellular composition of PBPC grafts obtained from healthy donors.

Rationale for allogeneic peripheral blood progenitor cell transplantation (PBPCT)

The possible advantages of unmanipulated allogeneic PBPCT instead of bone marrow transplantation (BMT) for the donor include that the risks and discomfort of the surgical procedure as well as general anaesthesia can be avoided, and that harvesting may be performed in an outpatient setting. Disadvantages for the donor comprise the exposition to haematopoietic growth factors and the need for undergoing leukapheresis with its associated risks. The recipient may experience a more rapid recovery of haematopoiesis and of the immune system, which should reduce treatment-related morbidity, facilitate earlier discharge from hospital, and decrease costs [4,5].

Safety issues

Successful harvesting of PBPC from healthy individuals requires mobilization with haematopoietic growth factors. Granulocyte colony-stimulating factor (G-CSF) is routinely used for this purpose because it is the safest among the agents available for PBPC priming. The predominant side effect of G-CSF is bone pain, which occurs in the vast majority of donors. In addition, 10-30% of healthy individuals treated with G-CSF suffer from symptoms such as headache, fatigue, and nausea [6-8].

G-CSF results in a rapid and dose-dependent leukocytosis (up to $50\text{-}70\times10^9$/L with 10 μg/kg) but has no immediate effect on haemoglobin levels and platelet counts [6,9]. However, some investigators have observed a delayed moderate decrease of platelets which can occur 6-9 days after start of G-CSF administration [6]. Since leukapheresis causes additional thrombocyte losses, platelet counts as low as 33×10^9/L have been observed in donors of allogeneic PBPC [7,9,10]. After G-CSF is stopped, a transient mild neutropenia can occur, which might be due to the inhibitory activity of other cytokines involved in the regulation of granulopoiesis or to suppression of endogeneous G-CSF production [11].

G-CSF has been administered safely to a large number of healthy subjects such as granulocyte donors and PBPC donors [7,9,12]. With the longest follow-up being more than five years, no case of late adverse events has been reported to date, and BM analysis of normal donors who received G-CSF 5 years earlier showed no evidence of morphological or cytogenetic abnormalities [13]. Even though G-CSF can stimulate leukemic blasts under certain conditions *in vitro*, there is no evidence that G-CSF exerts leukemogenic effects *in vivo* [14,15]. It is noteworthy that strongly elevated G-CSF levels also occur due to endogenous release of G-CSF, e.g. during severe infections [16]. Nevertheless, long-term adverse effects cannot be ruled out definitely at this point of time.

The risks of leukapheresis are generally low. Among 348 patients from the pooled data of 12 studies, one case of myocardial infarction shortly after leukapheresis for PBPC collection has been reported, and two other donors had angina pectoris-like symptoms during leukapheresis [17]. In addition, some donors complained of dysaesthesia during leukapheresis, which was severe in two cases [18, 19]. These symptoms were probably due to a transient hypocalcaemia induced by ACD-A used for anticoagulation during the separation. Approximately 10% of the donors needed a central venous blood flow which was complicated by a pneumothorax on 2 of 52 occasions [20,21]. In conclusion, leukapheresis is not a trivial procedure without any risk, but appropriate selection of donors (i.e. exclusion of individuals with cardiovascular risk factors or poor peripheral veins) should help to avoid serious complications. Weighed against the complications associated with BM harvesting under general anaesthesia [22] , however, the risks of G-CSF priming and leukapheresis in healthy donors seem to be by no means unacceptable.

PBPC collection

An adequate stem cell yield can be achieved with minimum collection efforts if the harvesting procedure is scheduled properly. The peak of CD34+ cells in the peripheral blood usually occurs on day 5 after the start of G-CSF administration [7-9], which is, thus, the optimum day for commencing leukapheresis. The mobilization efficacy of G-CSF appears to be dose-dependent [7,8,22]. Mobilization with 10-16 μg/kg allows harvesting of sufficient numbers of CD34+ cells with 1-2 leukapheresis procedures in the vast majority of donors. Among 35 donors of allogeneic PBPC primed with 10 μg/kg filgrastim, we observed only one individual yielding less than 1×10^6/kg CD34+ cells per 10L collection volume, while 43% reached the target dose of 4×106/kg with a single leukapheresis.

Cellular composition of mobilized PBPC grafts

G-CSF-mobilized PBPC from healthy donors comprise primitive as well as lineage-restricted progenitor cells [18]. In-vitro and *in-vivo* studies have demonstrated that all cells necessary for restoring complete haematopoiesis are present in allogeneic PBPC grafts[23,24].

Unmanipulated PBPC harvests obtained from healthy individuals contain about one log more T cells than allogeneic marrow grafts [9,12]. This is not only important with regard to potential GvH and GvL activities, but has also implications for the reconstitution of the immune system post transplant. Preliminary data indicate that the recovery of T cell numbers and function after allogeneic PBPCT is much faster than after BMT [25].

The T cells present in PBPC grafts are not only quantitatively but also qualitatively different from marrow T cells: It has been demonstrated in mice that the T cells contained in G-CSF-mobilized PBPC grafts express predominantly the type-2 cytokine pattern, which are believed to be capable of modulating acute GvH reactions after allogeneic BMT. In peripheral blood T cells of mice not exposed to G-CSF shows the type-1 pattern [26]. In comparison to marrow grafts, PBPC harvests are also characterized by an increased proportion of NK cells [9], which may be important for GvL activities [27].

Engraftment after allogeneic PBPCT

The engraftment seen after allogeneic primary transplantation of PBPC is complete and durable [28-30]. The speed of haematopoietic recovery after allogeneic PBPCT, however, is much more variable than it usually is after syngeneic or autologous transplantation. The reasons for this observation may include the genetic difference between graft and recipient. GvHD, veno-occlusive disease (VOD), viral infections, and the use of methotrexate for prophylaxis of GvHD. Nevertheless, the reconstitution of haematopoiesis after allogeneic PBPCT seems to be more rapid than after BMT. In four recent studies comprising a total of 147 patients, the median duration to achieve a neutophil count of more than 0.5×10^9/L and a platelet count of more than 20×10^9/L ranged from 14 to 15 days and from 10 to 16 days, respectively [10,19,31,32].

GvHD and GvL reactivity

To date there is no evidence for a significant difference between PBPCT and BMT with regard to acute GvHD. In the four larger series mentioned earlier [10, 19,31,32] grade II-IV disease was observed in 38-66% of patients, and grade III-IV in 13-25%, which is similar to the range that would be expected for allogeneic BMT. Limited or extensive chronic GvHD occurred in 32% to 79% patients at risk. Since the vast majority of these patients were older or had other risk factors known to be associated with an increased incidence of chronic GvHD, definite conclusions on the impact of allogeneic PBPCT in comparison to BMT on chronic GvHD cannot be drawn.

With regard to GvL efficacy, preliminary data observed in patients with CML suggest that complete eradication of disease as revealed by bcr/abl PCR may occur more often after PBPCT than after BMT [33]. This is in accordance with our own experience obtained in a mouse model comparing the GvL activity of PBPC and BM allografts, respectively. In an MHC-matched setting, transplantation of unmanipulated PBPC into lethally irradiated recipients who had been contaminated with the B-lymphoblastic leukemia A20 resulted in a reduction of the relapse rate to 29%, which was significantly lower than the leukemia incidence observed after identical numbers of unmanipulated marrow cells (60%; $p<0.05$) [34].

T cell depletion

Successful attempts to manipulate allogeneic BM grafts for eliminating GvH-reactive cells were undertaken already in the seventies [35]. In the clinical situation, however, T cell depletion (TCD) of bone marrow grafts has been hampered by a dramatic rise in the incidence of engraftment failure and strongly increased relapse rates. PBPC may allow to avoid these problems because of the "unlimited" amounts of stem cells and GvH/GvL effector cells which can be harvested from mobilized blood. We have reported previously that 3-4 logs of T cells can be depleted from PBPC grafts by CD34+ selection [35]. Others have confirmed these data and used CD34+ selected PBPC grafts for clinical allotransplantation [37-39]. Surprisingly, acute GvHD occurred in a significant proportion of patients in spite of transplanting $<1\times10^5$/kg T cells. Thus, more vigorous TCD appears to be neccessary for preventing GvHD effectively. Double purging strategies can achieve TCD of >4 log and result in complete elimination of GvHD even in a haploidentical setting [40]. The incidence of graft failure was very low in these preliminary trials, indicating that the problem of non-engraftment can indeed be circumvented by the use of PBPC.

In summary, allogeneic PBPCT is a promising alternative to BMT. The ongoing randomized studies will prove if transplantation of unmanipulated allogeneic peripheral blood stem cells is superior to BMT in terms of donor convenience, engraftment, and overall survival. However, the main advantage of allogeneic PBPC over BM appears to be their perfect suitability for graft engineering, such as T cell depletion, ex-vivo expansion, or generation of GvL effector cells. "Tailored cell therapy" by designing an allograft matching the individual needs of the recipient with regard to progenitor cells, GvL effector cells, and cells with specific anti-infectious activity appears to be a serious possibility.

References

1. Dreger P, Suttorp M, Haferlach T, Schroyens W, Löffler H, Schmitz N. Allogeneic G-CSF-mobilised peripheral blood progenitor cells for treatment of engraftment failure after bone marrow transplantation. Blood 1993;81:1404-07.
2. Russell NH, Hunter A, Rogers S, Hanley J, Anderson D. Peripheral blood stem cells as an alternative to marrow for allogeneic transplantation. Lancet, 1993;341:1482-82.
3. Gratwohl A, Hermans J, Baldomero H. Blood and marrow transplantation in Europe. Bone Marrow Transpl, 1997;19(in press).
4. Schmitz N, Linch, DC, Dreger P, et al. Randomised trial of filgrastim-mobilised peripheral blood progenitor cell transplantation versus autologous bone-marrow transplantation in lymphoma patients. Lancet, 1996;347:353-57.
5. Smith TJ, Hillner BE, Schmitz N, et al. Economic analysis of a randomized trial to compare filgrastim-mobilized peripheral blood progenitor cell transplantation and autologous bone marrow transplantation in patients with Hodgkin and Non-Hodgkin lymphoma. J Clin Oncol 1997;15:5-10.

6. Stroncek DF, Clay ME, McCullough J. Experiences of normal individuals treated with granulocyte colony stimulating factor. Blood 1994;84(Suppl-1):541a(Abstr).
7. Bensinger WI, Buckner CD, Rowley S, Storb R, Appelbaum, FR. Treatment of normal donors with recombinant growth factors for transplantation of allogeneic blood stem cells. Bone Marrow Transpl, 1996;17(Suppl 2):S19-S21.
8. Grigg AP, Roberts AW, Raunow H, et al. Optimizing dose and scheduling of filgrastim (granulocyte colony-stimulating factor) for mobilization and collection of peripheral blood progenitor cells in normal volunteers. Blood 1995;86:4437-45.
9. Dreger P, Haferlach T, Eckstein V. G-CSF-mobilized peripheral blood progenitor cells for allogeneic transplantation: Safety, kinetics of mobilization, and composition of the graft. Brit J Haematol, 1994;87:609-13.
10. Azevedo WM., Aranha FJP, Gouvea JV, et al. Allogeneic transplantation with blood stem cells mobilized by rhG-CSF for haematological malignancies. Bone Marrow Transpl 1995;16:647-53.
11. Anderlini P, Przepiorka D, Seong D, Champlin R, Körbling M. Transient neutropenia in normal donors after G-CSF mobilization and stem cell apheresis. Brit J Haematol 1996;94:155-58.
12. Körbling M, Huh YO, Durett A, et al. Allogeneic blood stem cell transplantation: Peripheralization and yield of donor-derived primitive haematopoietic progenitor cells (CD34+ Thy-1) and lymphoid subsets, and possible predictors of engraftmcnt and graft-versus-host disease. Blood 1995;86:2842-48.
13. Sakamaki S, Matsunaga T, Hirayama Y, Kuga T. Nitzsy Y. Haematological study of healthy volunteers 5 years after G-CSF. Lancet. 1995;346:1432-33.
14. Kawase Y, Akashi M, Ohtsu H, Aoki Y, Akanuma A, Suzuki G. Effect of human recombinant granulocyte colony-stimulating factor on induction of myeloid leukemias by X-irradiation in mice. Blood 1993;82:2163-68.
15. Imashuku S, Hibi S, Nakajima F, et al. A review of 125 cases to determine the risk of myelodysplasia and leukemia in pediatric neutropenic patients after treatment with recombinant human granulocyte colony-stimulating factor. Blood 1994;84:2380-81.
16. Kawakami M, Tsutsumi H, Kumakawa T, et al.Levels of serum granulocyte colony-stimulating factor in patients with infections. Blood 1990;76:1962-64.
17. Dreger P, Glass B, Uharek L, Zeis M, Schmitz N. Allogeneic transplantation of mobilized peripheral blood progenitor cells: Towards tailored cell therapy. Int J Hematol 1997 (in press).
18. Dreger P, Oberböster K, Schmitz N. PBPC grafts from healthy donors: Analysis of CD34+ and CD3+ subpopulations. Bone Marrow Transpl 1996;17(Suppl 2): S22-S27.
19. Bacigalupo A, van Lint MT, Valbonesi M, et al. Thiotepa/cyclophosphamide followed by granulocyte colony-stimulating factor mobilized allogeneic peripheral blood cells in adults with advanced leukemia. Blood, 1960;88:353-57.
20. Urbano-Ispizua A, Solano C, Brunet S, et al. Allogeneic peripheral blood progenitor cell transplantation: Analysis of short-term engraftment and acute GvHD incidence in 33 cases. Bone Marrow Transpl 1996;18:35-40.
21. Russell JA, Luider J, Weaver M, et al.Collection of progenitor cells for allogeneic transplantation from peripheral blood of normal donors. Bone Marrow Transpl 1995; 15:111-15.
22. Buckner CD, Petersen FB, Bolonesi BA. Bone marrow donors. Forman SJ, Blume KG, Thomas ED (eds) Bone marrow transplantation. Blackwell Scientific Publications, Boston 1994:259
23. Harada M, Nagafuji K, Fujisaki T, et al. G-CSF-Induced mobilization of peripheral blood stem cells from healthy adults for allogeneic transplantation. J Haematother 1996;5:63-71.

24. Molineux G, Pojda .Z, Hampson LN, Lord BL, Dexter TM. Transplantation potential of peripheral blood stem cells induced by granulocytic colony-stimulating factor. Blood 1990;76:2153-158.
25. Ottinger HD Beelen DW, Scheulen B, Schaefer UW, Grosse-Wilde H. Improved immune reconstitution after allotransplantation of periphcral blood stem cells instead of bone marrow. Blood 1996;88:2775-79.
26. Pan L, Delmonte J, Jalonen CK, Ferrara JLM. Pretreatment of donor mice with granulocyte colony-stimulating factor polarizes donor T-lymphocytes toward type-2 cytokine production and reduces severity of experimental graft-versus-host disease. Blood 1995;86:4422-29.
27. Glass B, Uharek L, Zeis M, Löffler H, Müller-Ruchholtz W, Gassmann W. Graft-versus-leukemia activity can be predicted by natural cytotoxicity against leukemia cells. Brit J Haematol 1996;93:412-20.
28. Schmitz N, Dreger P, Suttorp M, et al. Primary transplantation of allogeneic peripheral blood progenitor cells mobilized by filgrastim (G-CSF). Blood 1995;85:1666-72.
29. Körbling M, Przepiorka D, Engel H, et al. Allogeneic blood stem cell transplantation for refractory leukemia and lymphoma: Potential advantage of blood over marrow allografts. Blood 1995;85:1659-65.
30. Bensinger WI, Weaver CH, Appelbaum FR, Buckner CD. Transplantation of allogeneic peripheral blood stem cells mobilized by recombinant human granulocyte colony-stimulating factor (rhG-CSF). Blood 1995; 85:1655-58.
31. Bensinger WI, Buckner CD, Storb R, Demirer T, Appelbaum FA. Transplantation of allogeneic peripheral blood stem cells. Bone Marrow Transpl 1996;17(Suppl 2): S56-S57.
32. Schmitz N, Bacigalupo A, Labopin M, et al. Transplantation of allogeneic peripheral blood progenitor cells: The EBMT experience. Bone Marrow Transpl 1996;17 (Suppl 2):S40-S46.
33. Elmaagacli AH, Beelen DW. Becks HW, et al. Molecular studies of chimerism and minimal residual disease after allogeneic peripheral blood progenitor cell or marrow transplantation. Ann Hematol, 1996;73(Suppl 2);84(Abstr).
34. Zeis M, Uharek L, Glass B, Steinmann J, Dreger P, Schmitz N. Superior graft-vs-leukemia effects after transplantation of murine allogeneic peripheral blood progenitor cells (PBSC) as compared to bone marrow. Blood 1996;88(Suppl 1):245a(Abstr).
35. Müller-Ruchholtz W, Wottge HU, Müller-Hermelink HK. Bone marrow transplantation across strong histocompatibility barriers by selective elimination of lymphoid cells in bone marrow. Transplant Proc1976;8:537-41.
36. Dreger P, Viehmann K, Steinmann J. G-CSF-mobilised peripheral blood progenitor cells for allogeneic transplantation: Comparison of T cell depletion strategies using different CD34+ selection systems or CAMPATH-1. Exp Hematol 1995;23:147-154.
37. Bensinger WI, Buckner CD, Rowley S, Demirer T, Storb R, Appelbaum FA. Transplantation of allogeneic CD34+ peripheral blood stem cells (PBSC) in patients with advanced haematologic malignancy. Bone Marrow Transpl 1996;17(Suppl 2): S38-S39.
38. Corringham RET, Ho AD. Rapid and sustained allogeneic transplantation using immunoselected CD34+-selected peripheral blood progenitor cells mobilized by recombinant granulocyte-and granulocyte-macrophage colony-stimulating factors. Blood 1995;86:2052-54.
39. Link H, Arseniev L, Bähre O, Kadar JG, Diedrich.H, Poliwoda H. Transplantation of allogeneic CD34+ blood cells. Blood 1995:87.4903-09.
40. Martelli MF, Aversa F, Velardi A, et al. New tools for crossing the HLA barrier: Fludarabine and megadose stem cell transplants. Blood 1996:8.8(Suppl 1)484a(Abstr).

DISCUSSION

N.M. Heddle and H.J.C. de Wit – moderators

C.Th. Smit Sibinga (Groningen, NL): Dr. Muylle, what do we have in our hands in terms if standardisation of cytokine assays and what is the variation coefficient of these assays, because you showed quite a bit of variation in the cytokine outcome of the tests in various kits. So, what is the variation coefficient, how reliable are they and how do you standardise?

Dr. Fujihara, how do the ELISA assays relate to the bio-assays, because what you are testing in the ELISA is slightly different from what you do when you apply a bio-assay. It may be on the one hand side a little more sensitive, a little more specific, but does it relate to the functionality of the cytokines, which you tested in your bio-assays and not so much in your ELISA.

A final question to both of you. What do we know about the rate of cytokine production of white cells under normal standard physiological conditions. So not during storage of platelets under non-physiological conditions, because that is absolutely different. What is the rate of production in the normal circulating cell. Do we know anything about that?

M. Fujihara (Sapporo, J): ELISA assays may not completely relate to the functionality of cytokines, because ELISA detects active molecules as well as precursor proteins, denatured or degraded material. In addition, the difference between ELISA result and bio-assay result may be due to the presence of interfering molecules, which I talked about. Particularly the presence of soluble cytokine receptor may contribute to the discrepancy between two assays. In the case of TNF-α, the soluble TNF-α receptor inhibits biological activity. But if you assay TNF-α by ELISA you cannot distinguish the free TNF-α from TNF-α which is bound to the soluble TNF-α receptor. In the case of IL-6 the soluble IL-6 receptor can synergise IL-6. So, I think it is necessary to use more than one method to confirm cytokine level in a particular situation.

L. Muylle (Edegem, B): There is indeed a large variation in the cytokine outcome of the tests in different kits. This may be caused by several interfering factors as explained by Dr. Fujihara. However, the coefficient variation of a given ELISA test kit is in the range of 1-7% (intra-assay) and 5-13% (interassay). The difficulty is to recognise and measure the bioactive molecules. Therefore, it is advisable to select test kits using neutralising (binding to active sites) monoclonal antibodies. In a study international standards have been used to perform calibration curves for all the ELISA kits used[1]. The coefficients of variation were then significantly improved for measurements of IL-6 and IL-8 but not for IL-1 and TNF-α. However, none of the kits gave similar values for individual samples. Therefore, further work is required and the choice of the ELISA kit and the use of the same reagents throughout a given study are important.

Data exist about the production of cytokines under in vitro conditions. However, I am not aware of data concerning the rate of production in the normal circulating cell.

H.J.C. de Wit (Leeuwarden, NL): Could it also be that the processing done by the different researchers in different parts of the world using different materials, different volumes of whole blood is a factor? That could be very contributional to the differences found in IL-8, IL-6 at the end.

L. Muylle: Yes, the leukocyte content could be different and the time the samples are taken also.There is a need to define more accurately what is meant by day 0, day 1 or day 5. Are samples always taken at the same time of the day?

H.J.C. de Wit: And the standardisation of production methods?

L. Muylle: Yes, if you want to compare, you have to standardise everything.

C.Th. Smit Sibinga: A final comment. So, by all means, what you observe ex vivo in a platelet concentrate reflects more or less a natural production all be it under not so physiological circumstances. That means that there will be an increase in the level, rather than to speak of a high level. High compares to the starting point. However, what you observe reflects the normal activity of lymphocytes to produce cytokines.

L. Muylle: Well, what we observe reflects the production of cytokines by leukocytes, that are most probably activated.

C.Th. Smit Sibinga: Correct, it reflects the production of cytokines, which is a normal function of lymphocytes. So when you start with a product which you just have harvested and then measure in the time, you measure actually the activity, which is grossly the normal activity of lymphocytes. So what you end up with reflects more or less an accumulation of normal production of cytokines and maybe some extra stimulation due to interaction with the plastics and so forth.

H.J.C. de Wit: But there is no normal elimination.

---

1. Ledur A, Fitting C, David B. Hamberger Chr, Cavailon JM. Variable estimates of cytokine levels produced by commercial ELISA kits: results using international cytokine standards. J Immunol Methods 1995;186:171-79.

C.Th. Smit Sibinga: That is true, but there is degradation as well.

L. Muylle: Yes, that is true. In addition, if you contaminate a platelet concentrate with bacteria you will have a much higher response.

B. Löwenberg (Rotterdam, NL): A question along the same line. I was really surprised to see that all these studies dealt with a limited number of cytokines. Today we know of various other cytokines that are actively produced by monocytes and lymphocytes following specific inductions. These were not included in the analysis. What about G-CSF and various other cytokines; did anyone look at those?

A second question is; Dr. Heddle is going to discuss the relationships to morbidity, but what about in vivo levels. When these products with elevated concentrations of cytokines are transfused, is there any increase in vivo of the serum levels of these cytokines, in other words is there a measurable transfer? Could you perhaps comment on these questions?

L. Muylle: In answer to your second question, we have not yet measured the effect of transfusing high levels of cytokines into a patient to see if the cytokine level increases in the patient. One can anticipate that this will be so, but only for a very short time. When you measure cytokine levels after intravenous injection of high doses of human cytokines very short peaks are observed; so if you infuse something that is 100 times less I wonder if any effect could be seen.

B. Löwenberg: That was my question, but this has apparently not been addressed.

N.M. Heddle (Hamilton, C): Nobody in our group has addressed that either, but I know there is one report in the literature. I believe it was published as a letter to the editor in Transfusion by Ron Sacher's group at Georgetown University Medical Centre[1] and presented at an ASH meeting[2]. They actually looked at a number of patients (over 40 patients), who received transfusions. IL-6 was measured post transfusion and they found that the patients who did have reactions had higher levels of IL-6 compared to the control group, but there was no mention in the publications that they actually measured IL-6 in the blood products given. So, whether the increase was actually passive transfer of IL-6 or in vivo generation is unclear. I think that studies like that would definitely be very useful in helping to sort this out.

J. Kadar (Hannover, D): We just recently finished a pilot study dealing with the core problem of leukocyte reduction; production of leukocyte reduced platelet con-

---

1. Sacher RA, Boyle L, Freter CE. High circulating interleukin levels associated with acute transfusion reactions: cause or effect? (letter) Transfusion 1993;33:962.
2. Boyle L, McLesky S, Freter C, Sacher RA. High circulating interleukin-6 levels associated with acute transfusion reaction. Cause or effect? Blood 1994;84(Suppl):463a.

centrates without using filters; the storage properties of these concentrates including the measurement of IL-6 and IL-8 as well as the IL-6 and IL-8 levels after transfusion. This pilot study included post bone marrow transplantation patients; in the first 40 patients we did not observe any correlation between the IL-6 and IL-8 levels in the concentrate and the post transplant IL-6 and IL-8 levels. There was no change within 1 hour of IL-6 and IL-8 in the patients. If the IL-6 was higher than normal because of GvH or post transplant clinical problems, there was also no change in the level, maybe because the transfusion was not contaminated with any leukocytes

B. Löwenberg: Dr. Rill and Dr. Mertelsmann what is the current strategy that you are exploring to increase the efficiency of gene transfer into haematopoietic stem cells; a problem that both of you recognised in your presentation. Dr. Rill mentioned the various cytokines that are going to be used, but none of you was very specific on this point. Could you perhaps elaborate on that and give your views?

D.R. Rill (Memphis, TN, USA): We are currently looking at several options. We have done much pre-clinical work with use of cytokine combinations that is pretty well published, mostly IL-1 data , IL-3, IL-6 and stem cell factor to increase the number of CD34 cells in cycle[1]. Unfortunately, in our circumstances it tends to push the cells a little farther into commitment than we desire them to be for vector gene transfer. One approach that we are looking at heavily is using a combination of vector systems.We are currently evaluating using the adenovirus to carry retroviral receptors. We are getting very good transfer efficiency with adenoviral vectors running between 80 and 85% in CD34 cells, but we do not get any integration. So, we are looking at using adenoviral/ retroviral receptor to the CD34 cell and then to carry in a gene of interest with a retroviral vector in a very early to middle stage. We are trying several possibilities.

R. Mertelsmann (Freiburg, D): With respect to delivering cytokines, of course, gene transfer is not the real problem, because we use clonally selected cells. So you just pick the cells that make the amount of cytokine that you are looking for. It is more a question of vector design, the type of promoter you use. So, using clonally selected fibroblast gene transfer is not the problem. For gene transfer into CD34 haematopoietic stem cells we use a pseudo-typed vector. We developed a serum free medium containing SCF FLT 3 ligand and interleukin 3 which are based on the data that Dr. Henschler[2] generated expanding long term culture initiating cells by about a factor 5 while pushing cells into cycle. The data that we have sofar look very promising, and this might be a major step in the right direction.

B. Löwenberg: How sure can we be that the lack of cell cycling really is the major determinant of the inability of gene transfer of haemotopoietic cells.

---

1. Personal communication.
2. Unpublished.

R. Mertelsmann: It certainly applies to retroviruses.

B. Löwenberg: Yes, but still there is to explain the difference between the murine and the human system. On both sides there is of course a limited fraction of primitive stem cells that is actively cycling and would be difficult to transduce, but what is your opinion about other vectors that are more specific to the properties of the stem cell for instance surface properties. And how would targeting be an important tool in developing the efficiency. Can you comment?

R. Mertelsmann: Many people are working on that and we looked at cell mediated gene transfer together with the group in Vienna and that was not very successful. I think there was a paper in Blood using adenoviral vector[1]. I do not recall which group it was. So, I think the field is wide open. Retroviruses sofar have the advantage that they do work, that they are clinically safe as far as we know. In my opinion it is still the best bet, so we focus rather on changing the culture conditions to generate cells, which are optimally suited to be gene transduced by retroviruses. That is our approach.

D.C. Dale (Seattle, WA, USA): Dr. Mertelsmann, have you been successful in getting long term expression of the haematopoietic growth factors from fibroblasts. If so, how long can you do that.

R. Mertelsmann: That is, of course, the central problem. If the cells continue to grow, you get long term gene expression in vivo. That is I think very clear and that is what other people also have seen. In the human situation there is always some residual baseline gene expression. So, one approach is to increase gene expression by a factor of thousand of baseline expression that will yield sufficient product to be therapeutically efficacious. That is the route that we are pursuing. Generate the vector that is a thousand times better and what is left after methylation or whatever changes occur, is enough to have a therapeutically active product. That is our strategy. In non-immunosuppressed situations you clearly have the problem of immune responses, so repeated infections. In the short term expression situation after chemotherapy you have two advantages. You have immunosuppression based on the cytokine plus you only need short term gene expression and here we have been able in the murine model to use repeated injections of these irradiated cytokine producing cells, which were therapeutically active. But consistent long term high level expressions still are an illusive project.

C.Th. Smit Sibinga: Dr. Dreger, the step towards allogeneic peripheral blood stem cells by stimulating donors, of course, was a very obvious one and has been discussed several times. It is slightly out of the scope of this symposium, but I

1. Watanabe T, Kuszynski C, Ino K, et al. Gene transfer into human bone marrow haematopoietic cells mediated by adenovirus vectors. Blood 1996;87:5032-39.

would like to have your comments on the alternative which is now rapidly coming up: using allogeneic cord or placental stem cells, which have the advantage of a vast access, the advantage of less expression of specifically class II antigens on their surface and providing therefor less severe and less evident GvHD. Don't you think we are going that way now and therefor re-evaluate the approach of stimulating donors?

P. Dreger (Kiel, D): Maybe that cord blood transplantations will become an important alternative or perhaps the main source of stem cells in the future. I think at the present time there is too few data available to claim that at this time you can have a reasonable alternative, when using cord blood cells instead of bone marrow or peripheral blood progenitor cells, because most of the data published on cord blood cells in the clinical situation related to children. So, I think there has to be some additional evidence to be shown that also adults can be transplanted safely with the smaller amount of stem cells, which are present in unexpanded cord blood donations. Maybe when we have some progress in cell expansion technologies, this will be different.

C.Th. Smit Sibinga: Agreed, the series are still limited although in a recent presentation Dr. Kurzberg reported already a substantial number of adult patients, that showed a remarkable recovery on much smaller dosages of cells[1]. So, there is evidence coming up. The time is still too early, I fully agree on that, but the question was more philosophical: do you think that it is going that way, because I think it is going that way.

P. Dreger: It may be that this will be the predominant source of stem cells in the future, but I think at the present time one should follow both directions studying peripheral blood progenitor cells as well as cord blood stem cells to have optimally designed grafts in the future. In particular with regards to graft versus leukaemia effects peripheral blood progenitor cells offer advantages because there are much more T-cells and much more effector cells you can deal with.

---

1. Kurzberg J, Laughlin M, Smith C et al. Placental umbilical cord blood: an alternative source for hemopoietic stem cells for bone marrow reconstitution in unrelated donor transplantation. Vox Sang 1996;70(Suppl 2):43(Abstr.).

III. ROLE AND APPLICATION OF CYTOKINES AND GROWTH FACTORS IN CLINICAL MEDICINE

CLINICAL RELEVANCE OF CYTOKINE LEVELS IN BLOOD PRODUCTS: EVIDENCE TO CORRELATE WITH MORBIDITY[1]

N.M. Heddle

Introduction

Complications associated with the infusion of blood and blood products are not uncommon. They can present as acute reactions occurring during, or within a few hours of the transfusion, or as delayed events, presenting days or possibly years later (Table 1). Patient morbidity is variable depending on the type of reaction and with some reactions mortality can occur [1,2].

Table 1. Summary of the acute and delayed reactions that can occur with blood transfusion.

Adverse effects of transfusion	
Acute reaction	Haemolysis
	Febrile non-haemolytic reactions
	Allergic reactions
	Anaphylaxis
	Transfusion related acute lung injury
	Metabolic complications
	Bacterial contamination
Delayed reactions	Alloimmunization
	Delayed haemolytic transfusion reactions
	Graft-versus-Host Disease
	Disease/Viral transmission
	Post transfusion purpura

Over the past few years the role of biological response modifiers (BRM) in causing or contributing to these adverse effects has been recognized. In some circumstances the BRM may be generated *in vivo* because of antigen-antibody incompatibilities between the donor's and recipient's bloods; however, in other situations

1. This manuscript was supported in part by grants from the Miles-CRC Research Fund and the Medical Research Council of Canada.

it has been postulated that the signs and symptoms associated with these reactions are caused by BRM present in the blood product [3]. When the product is transfused these substances cause the morbidity typical of these events. This manuscript will focus on clinical evidence that cytokines in blood products are a cause of transfusion associated morbidity.

Biological response modifiers in transfusion products

Laboratory studies have demonstrated the accumulation of a variety of biological response modifiers in platelet and red cell products during storage [4-9].

Platelet products

The concentration of pro-inflammatory cytokines such as interleukin-1β (IL-1β), interleukin-6 (IL-6), and tumour necrosis factor α (TNFα) all increase in platelet products prepared from platelet rich plasma during storage [4,7,9]. The concentrations of these cytokines after five days of platelet storage are related to the leukocyte concentration in the product. When the leukocyte concentration is reduced pre-storage to $\leq 10^6$ cells/product using filtration techniques, these cytokines are no longer detectable [7,9,10]. Pro-inflammatory cytokines are not usually detectable in stored platelets that have been prepared by the buffy coat technique [11]. This observation suggests that the threshold of leukoreduction needed to prevent detectable cytokine generation in platelet products during storage may be in the range of 10^7 to 10^8 leukocytes per product.

Chemokines such as interleukin-8 (IL-8) are also detectable in platelets prepared from platelet rich plasma, with concentrations approximately 10 to 15 times higher than those of the pro-inflammatory cytokines [6]. It has been postulated that IL-8 could play a role in transfusion related acute lung injury (TRALI) because of its chemotactic function for neutrophils, but IL-8 may also contribute to febrile non-haemolytic transfusion reactions (FNHTR) because of its activating activity. Other potential biological response modifiers that have been detected in stored platelet products include: complement fragments C3a and C4a [8,12]; lipids that are capable of priming neutrophil NADPH oxidase [5,13]; RANTES [14] and macrophage inflammatory protein (MIP-1) [15].

Red cell products

A number of biological response modifiers have also been detected in red cell concentrates after 42 days of storage; however, like the platelet products the presence of these substances appears to be influenced by the method of red cell preparation [16,17]. Red cells prepared following the removal of platelet rich plasma have detectable IL-1β and IL-8 after 42 days of storage; however, the concentrations of IL-8 are in the range of 100-200 pg/ml which is approximately ten times lower than the concentrations detectable in stored platelet products. IL-6 has not been detected in these products. IL-1β and IL-6 are not usually detected in red cell concentrates prepared by the buffy coat method. IL-8 is detectable in red cells prepared from buffy coats on day one of storage (range 8.3

pg/ml to 1071.2 pg/ml) but the levels appear to decrease over the 42 day storage period (range 8.1 to 407.2) [17]. It is possible that the centrifugation technique required for this method results in the release of IL-8 from cell surfaces, or from neutrophils and monocytes, with subsequent reabsorption of IL-8 to the red cell surface during the storage period [18]. The concentrations of cytokines in red cell concentrates are significantly lower than the levels seen in platelet products. This may be the result of storage conditions such as temperature and agitation as both of these variables have been shown to affect cytokine levels in stored platelet products [19]. Other biologic response modifiers detected in red cell concentrates include histamine[20] and lipid compounds [13].

Assessment of clinical evidence

Whenever a strong association is observed between an individual factor (i.e. cytokine) and a clinical event (i.e. a reaction to transfusion), it is tempting to postulate a cause/effect relationship; however, as noted in Figure 1 this may not always be logical or appropriate. Evidence to support an association between the cytokine levels in a blood product and the risk of a reaction can be examined by critically reviewing clinical data related to this issue. When reviewing this data it is important to recognize the strength and weakness of the data based on the methodologies that were used. It is well accepted that an experimental study using a randomized double blind design provides the strongest clinical evidence, followed by prospective cohort studies; then studies using case-control designs. Case reports

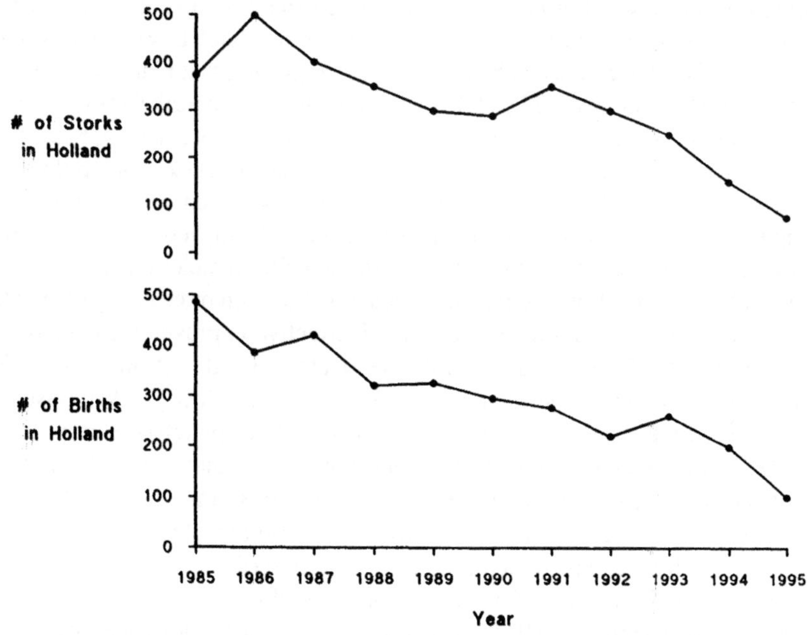

Figure 1. Graph showing the association between storks in Holland and birth rate to illustrate that a strong association does not always mean a cause-effect relationship.

and case series are good for hypothesis generating but should not be used for evidence based practice [21]. It is also important that the study be critically appraised using well recognized and established criteria to ensure the validity of the methodology used and the conclusions [22,23].

There are currently three types of reactions in which the passive transfusion of BRM in the blood product have been suggested as the responsible factors causing morbidity. These include: febrile non-haemolytic transfusion reactions, transfusion related acute lung injury and allergic (urticarial) reactions.

Febrile non-haemolytic transfusion reactions (FNHTRs)

Febrile non-haemolytic transfusion reactions to red cells were recognized and investigated in the late 1950's and early 1960's. These reactions were characterized by a rise in temperature of greater than 1 °C which was frequently accompanied by: chills; a cold sensation; rigors; discomfort; and occasionally nausea and headache. When these symptoms could not be explained by the patient's clinical condition, it was assumed that they were transfusion induced [24]. Laboratory investigations suggested that these reactions were immune mediated events caused by white cell antibodies in the patient's plasma that reacted with leukocytes present in the red cell product. The clinical observation that most reactions could be prevented by reducing the leukocyte concentration to a threshold of 5×10^{8} per product supported the proposed etiology of this event [25-28].

When platelet concentrates routinely became available in late 1960 and throughout the 1970's, it was noted that FNHTRs could also occur when this product was transfused. It was assumed that these reactions were also mediated by leukocyte antibodies. The frequency of FNHTRs to platelets was significantly higher than red cell reactions with several groups reporting that reactions occurred with 20% to 30% of transfused platelets compared to frequencies of 1% to 6% with red cell products [29-31]. In addition to this discrepancy in frequency, there were several other laboratory and clinical observations that suggested the etiology for platelet reactions could be different than the etiology of red cell reactions. For example, males who had not been previously transfused and were not sensitized to leukocyte antibodies, often had a reaction to their first platelet transfusion [31]; removal of leukocytes from the platelet product by filtration or centrifugation to the threshold of $<5\times10^{8}$ cells/product was often ineffective in preventing reactions to platelet products [29-31] and, several investigators noted a strong association between the risk of a reaction and the age of the platelet product [31,32]. Based on these observations it was hypothesized that FNHTRs to platelets were product-mediated being caused by biological response modifiers that accumulated in the supernatant plasma of the platelet product during the storage period. This new hypothesis led a number of investigators to look for biological response modifiers in platelet products as mentioned previously and described in more detail in the paper by Muylle [33]. Most of the investigations in this area have focused on the pro-inflammatory cytokines (IL-β, IL-6 and TNF), as these substances are known to be pyrogenic and capable of causing the symptoms typical of FNHTR.

Clinical evidence for product associated BRM and FNHTR to platelets

There are a number of clinical studies that provide evidence for a cause-effect relationship between febrile non-haemolytic transfusion reactions and the passive infusion of cytokines in platelet products. In two of these studies, cytokine levels were measured in the transfused platelet products to determine if there was a correlation between the cytokine level and a reaction. Muylle et al. [4] performed an observation study that involved a series of 45 platelet transfusions of which six of the transfusions were associated with reactions. They measured the concentrations of the pro-inflammatory cytokines (IL-1β, IL-6 and TNF) in each transfused product, and found that the levels were significantly higher in the six platelet products associated with reactions compared to the 39 platelet products that were not associated with adverse effects.

Our laboratory used a different approach to investigate the possibility that biological response modifiers (ie: possibly cytokines) were the cause of FNHTRs to platelets [9]. Before transfusion, each platelet product was centrifuged to separate the supernatant plasma from the cellular component. Each portion of the product (plasma and cells) was transfused to the patient in random order and the patient was monitored for clinical evidence of a reaction. This approach was based on the assumption that a reaction caused by passive infusion of biological response modifiers would occur when the plasma portion of the product was infused; whereas, a reaction caused by leukocyte antibodies would be associated with the cellular portion of the product. The majority of reactions (58.8%), and the severest reactions (ie: severe chills and rigors) occurred when the plasma portion of the platelet product was transfused; however, 15.8% (6/34) of reactions were associated with only the cellular portion and 18.6% (8/34) of the reactions occurred to both portions of the product. These observations suggest that the cause of FNHTR may be multifactorial; however, the data strongly supports the hypothesis that biological response modifiers in the supernatant plasma are the cause of most FNHTR to platelets. Because of the ability of pro-inflammatory cytokines to cause fever, IL-1β and IL-6 were measured in each of the plasma supernatants transfused. The results were consistent with the Belgium report demonstrating a strong association between reactions and high cytokine levels. Although the association between FNHTR and cytokine levels in the platelet products have been reported in these two studies, one of the unanswered questions is whether the pro-inflammatory cytokines are the only agents responsible for these events, or whether other biological response modifiers in the platelet product could also play a role. As mentioned previously, there appears to be a number of biological response modifiers other than cytokines that are generated in platelet products during storage; hence, their potential contribution to these reactions cannot be excluded.

If one assumes that the BRM produced during storage are the predominate cause of FNHTRs, then interventions to prevent these reactions should focus on removing these substances before transfusion, or preventing the formation of these substances during the storage period [34].

Table 2. Possible techniques for removing or preventing biological responses modifiers (BRM) from accumulating in platelet products during storage.

Removing BRM from platelets	Plasma removal by centrifugation Filtration/adherence
Preventing accumulation of BRM in platelets	Leukoduction pre-storage Storage in a plasma free preservative solution Decreasing the storage interval

The various techniques for preventing or removing BRM before transfusion are listed in Table 2. Removal of BRMs can easily be accomplished by centrifugation of the product followed by removal of the plasma supernatant [9]. Preliminary data has shown that some BRM such as C3a, C4a and IL-8 can also be removed by filtration; however, current filters seem to have no effect on the removal of the pro-inflammatory cytokines [35-37]. There are several techniques that can be used to prevent or decrease the accumulation of BRM in platelets during storage. Reducing the storage interval to three days will result in lower cytokine concentrations [4,7,9]; however, this approach increases the demand for donor recruitment to meet the utilization needs; thus, in some areas this approach may not be feasible. The accumulation of some BRM (C3a, C4a) could be prevented by storing the platelet product in a plasma-free platelet storage solution as the accumulation of complement fragments results from an interaction between the plasma present in the product and the plastic surface of the storage bag [8,38,39]. An alternative approach which has been shown to prevent cytokine generation is pre-storage leukoreduction as the pro-inflammatory cytokines are derived from the leukocytes present in the platelet product [7,9,10].

The threshold of leukoreduction required to prevent cytokine accumulation appears to be in the range of 10^7 to 10^8 leukocytes per pooled product, as platelets prepared by the buffy coat technique have minimal or no cytokines detectable after five days of storage [11,17]. Leukoreduction by filtration, which results in less than or equal to 10^6 leukocytes per product also prevents cytokine accumulation [7,9]; however, based on the buffy coat data, this level of leukoreduction appears to be well below the required threshold. Leukoreduction will only prevent the accumulation of BRMs that are leukocyte derived (IL-1β, IL-6, TNF and IL-8), but will have no effect on the accumulation of non-leukocyte derived BRMs such as complement fragments C3a and C4a [8] and the lipids that are capable of priming neutrophils [5].

There have been a number of published studies that have investigated the frequency of FNHTRs following the transfusion of various types of leukoreduced platelet and red cell products (Tables 3 and 4). These studies provide indirect support for the association between BRM and FNHTRs, and also provide evidence that the biological response modifiers responsible for these reactions are leukocyte derived. The methodological design and the results from each of these studies is summarized below:

Table 3. Summary of the frequencies of reactions to platelets in clinical studies.

Study	Platelet product	Method of preparation	Filtration	Leukocytes transfused (mean)	Frequency of reaction
Muylle et al. [4]	RD[1)] (pool 8)	PRP[2)]	PL50 (bedside) post-storage	–	13.3 (6/45)
Oksanen et al. [40]	RD	PRP	–	–	50 (23/46)
	RD (pool 4)	PRP	Imugard IG-500®[4)] (post-storage)	0.04×10^6	22 (5/22)
	RD (pool 4)	BC[3)]	Imugard IG-500® (pre-storage)	0.008×10^6	4 (2/50)
	RD (pool 4)	BC	Imugard IG-500® (post-storage)	0.048×10^6	6 (2/36)
Anderson et al. [41]	SDAP[5)]	2997 COBE	–	6.9×10^9	2.1 (51/2429)
	SDAP	CS-3000 [Isoradial]	–	3.5×10^9	3.5 (120/3434)
	SDAP	V50	–	8.3×10^8	2.4 (3/125)
	SDAP	COBE SPECTRA	–	5.0×10^5	
Dzieckowski et al. [42]	SDAP	COBE SPECTRA CS-3000 Plus	–[6)]	$<0.5 \times 10^6$ [7)]	1.6 (82/5197)
Federowicz et al. [43]	SDAP[8)]	COBE SPECTRA CS-3000 Plus	–[9)]	$<0.5 \times 10^6$	1.7 (59/3405)
Bishop et al. [45]	RD	PRP	–	–	17.1 (20/117)
	RD	BC	–	–	4.1 (7/168)
	SDAP	–	–	–	3.6 (6/169)

1) Random donor platelets; 2) Platelet rich plasma; 3) Buffy coat; 4) Filtered within 72 hours of preparation; 5) Apheresis platelets; 6) Patients having 2 reactions to SDAP received products filtered at the bedside (PL50); 7) 94% of products had leukocyte counts below this level; 8) SDAP with $>0.5 \times 10^6$ leukocytes were filtered (LRF6); 9) Patients having 2 reactions to SDAP received products filtered in the laboratory (LRF6).

Table 4. Summary of the frequency of FNHTR to pre-storage and post-storage leukoreduced red cells reported in two studies from the Dana Farber Cancer Centre, Boston, MA.

Study	**Platelet product**	**Method of preparation**	**Method of leukoreduction**	**Mean leukocyte concentration**	**Frequency of reaction**
Dzieckowski et al.[42]	RCC [1)]	Adsol (AS-1)	RC50 [2)] (post-storage) or Frozen deglycerolized	–	2.2 (152/7080)
Federowicz et al. [43]	RCC	Adsol (AS-1)	BP4F (pre-storage)	1.3×10^{5}	1.1 (59/5412)

1) RCC - red cell concentrate; 2) 91% (6447/7080) of the RCC were filtered and 9% (633/7080) were frozen and deglycerolized.

Oksanen et al. (1994) [40]

This is a prospective study using a crossover design to compare the frequency of FNHTRs to platelet products prepared by the buffy coat technique that were either leukoreduced pre-storage or post-storage using an Imugard IG-500 filter (Terumo, Japan). There was no statistically significant difference in the frequency of reactions to the two types of platelet products (4% pre-storage leukoreduction versus 6% with post-storage leukoreduction). These results also were compared to retrospective data from a non-randomized study where patients had received either standard platelet products prepared by the PRP technique or leukoreduced platelets from PRP that were filtered within 72 hours of preparation. The frequency of reactions to standard platelets was 50% (23/46). Fewer reactions occurred with the platelet products prepared from PRP that were leukoreduced by filtration (22%); however, the difference was not statistically significant. Both PRP product types had a significantly higher frequency of reaction than the platelets prepared by the buffy coat technique. The results from this study supports the concept that the BRM that may cause platelet reactions are leukocyte derived, and suggests that the level of leukocyte reduction achieved with the buffy coat technique is adequate to significantly reduce most platelet reactions.

The next three studies were all reported from the Dana Farber Cancer Institute in Boston over a five year interval.

Anderson et al. (1991) [41]

The frequency of reactions to four different types of apheresis platelet products was investigated in this study. Platelets were collected using the following equipment: the COBE 2997 containing a mean of 6.9×10^9 leukocytes per product; the CS-3000 [Isoradial] and the V50 (Haemonetics, Braintree, MA) containing 3.5×10^9 leukocytes and 8.3×10^8 leukocytes respectively; and the COBE Spectra (COBE BCT, Lakewood, CO). Platelet products prepared using the COBE SPECTRA had the lowest level of leukocyte contamination with a mean level of 5.0×10^5 leukocytes per product. The frequencies of reactions to these four products were 2.1%, 3.5%, 2.4% and 1.5% respectively.

Dzieczkowski et al. (1995) [42]

The second study utilized a prospective observational design documenting the frequency of FNHTR in 911 patients who received 7,080 leukoreduced red cells and 5,197 single donor apheresis platelets. Red cell concentrates were prepared from whole blood collected into Adsol (AS-1). The leukocytes were removed by freezing and deglycerolization, or by using a RC50 bedside filter (Pall Biomedical Products, Glen Cove, NY). The apheresis platelets were collected on either the COBE Spectra or the CS3000 Plus (Fenwal Laboratories, Deerfield, IL) and had less than 5×10^6 leukocytes/ product in 94% of the products. If a patient had two FNHTR to the single donor apheresis product the platelets were then filtered at the bedside using a PL50 filter (Pall Biomedical Products, Glen Cove, NY). Reactions occurred in 14.7% (134/911) of the patients transfused. The frequency of FNHTR to red cells was 2.15% compared with 1.58% to the apheresis platelets.

Federowicz et al. (1996) [43]

This follow-up study from the same centre compared the frequency of reactions to red cell and platelet products that were leukoreduced pre-storage to products leukoreduced post-storage (at the time of transfusion). The pre-storage leukoreduced red cells were prepared from whole blood collected in Adsol (AS-1) then filtered with a BPF4 filter ($<1.3\times10^5$ leukocytes/product) one to two days after collection. The single donor platelets were collected using the same apheresis technology as the previous study which resulted in $<5\times10^6$ leukocytes in 94% of the products. Products exceeding this threshold were filtered in the laboratory using a LRF6 platelet filter. As with the previous study, once a patient had two FNHTR to the single donor apheresis platelets, the product was also filtered post-storage using a LRF6 laboratory filter. The results of this observational study were compared with the data collected earlier by Dzieczkowski et al [42]. Pre-storage leukoreduction of red cell concentrates resulted in a significant decrease in FNHTR. The frequency of reactions to the pre-storage leukoreduced red cell product was 1.1% which was 50% lower than the frequency of reactions to the post-storage leukoreduced product (2.2%). The frequency of FNHTR to platelets was 1.7% which was not significantly different from the frequency of reactions published earlier (1.6%); however, with both of these apheresis products the threshold of contaminating leukocytes was usually less than 0.5×10^6 leukocytes; thus, they could both be considered pre-storage leukoreduced.

Muir et al. (1995) [44]

Records from 19 haematology/oncology patients were retrospectively reviewed to determine the frequency of FNHTRs to platelets that were leukoreduced pre- and post-storage. The results showed that a patient had a 6.1-fold greater chance of a reaction with platelets leukoreduced post-storage compared to the pre-storage leukoreduced products. The frequency of reactions with the pre-storage leukoreduced product was 0.8% compared to 4.8% with post-storage leukoreduction. To date this study has only been published as an abstract.

Bishop et al. (1995) [45]

Patients in this study were randomized to receive platelets prepared from PRP, random donor platelets prepared from buffy coats, or single donor platelets collected on the COBE Spectra. The outcome measures included a comparison of one and 24 hour post-transfusion corrected count increments (CCI), and the frequency of reactions to the three product types. There was no difference in the CCI results at 24 hours; however, the 1 hour CCI was significantly higher with the apheresis product. The single donor apheresis platelets and the platelets prepared from buffy coats were associated with 3.6% and 4.1% reactions respectively. The frequency of reactions to the random donor product was significantly higher at 17.1%. The mean leukocyte counts on the three product types were not provided. The authors concluded that pre-storage leukoreduction to a threshold of $\leq 1\times10^7$ per product significantly reduces the frequency of FNHTRs.

Sacher et al. (1993) [46]

This is the only study in which IL-6 levels were measured *in vivo* pre- and post-transfusion in a group of 42 patients. Acute transfusion reactions occurred in 26 patients. The mean IL-6 level pre-transfusion in these patients was 35.7 pg/ml and rose to a mean of 134.8 pg/ml post-transfusion. The control group of 16 patients who did not experience acute reactions did not have a significant increase in IL-6 with a mean pre-transfusion level of 10 pg/ml which rose to 14.3 pg/ml post-transfusion. The concentration of IL-6 was not measured in the transfused blood products; hence, it is impossible to determine whether the detectable IL-6 was passively transfused or due to *in vivo* generation of IL-6 from the donor's or recipient's leukocytes. Additional studies that measure *in vivo* cytokines pre- and post-transfusion and cytokines in the transfused blood product would be useful to elucidate the role of passively transfused cytokines in blood products as a cause of FNHTRs.

What conclusion can be drawn from these studies that support or refute the cause-effect relationship between FNHTR to platelets and cytokines present in the blood product?

There are several observations that support the cause-effect relationship:

1. Random donor platelets prepared using the PRP technique appear to be associated with a higher frequency of FNHTR than platelets prepared from buffy coats (Figure 2). This observation supports the cause-effect relationship as the buffy

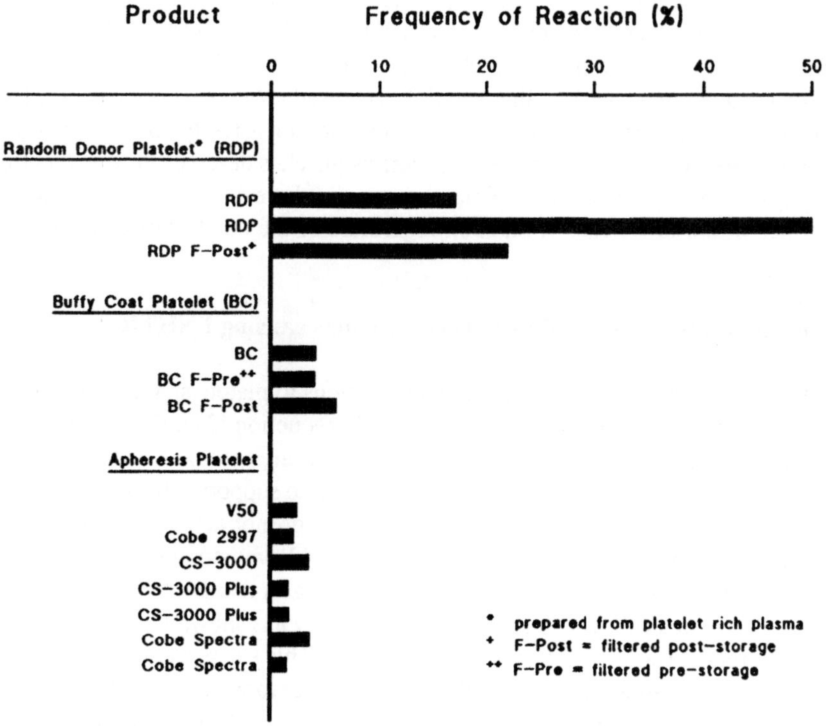

Figure 2. Frequency of FNHTR to platelets based on the product type.

coat platelets contain one to two logs fewer leukocytes per product than the product prepared from PRP. Laboratory studies have shown that this one to two log level of leukoreduction is sufficient to prevent cytokines (IL-1β, IL-6 and TNF) and chemokines (IL-8) from accumulating to any significant levels in the buffy coat products.

2. Pre-storage leukoreduced apheresis platelet products appear to be associated with a lower frequency of FNHTR (1.7%) than apheresis platelets that contained 10^9 leukocytes per product (reported frequencies of 2.1% to 3.5%). This also supports the BRM theory.

There are several additional observations which do not add additional support for the cause-effect relationship but instead raise questions regarding other mechanisms that may be responsible for a small percentage of FNHTR as these reactions still occur with 2% to 4% of platelet transfusions even when the platelet product is leukoreduced to a threshold of 10^6 per product prior to storage. It is possible that patients with potent leukocyte antibodies may react to platelet products even when the leukocyte concentration is at a low threshold. Alternatively, the accumulation of biological response modifiers other than cytokines may be responsible for these residual reactions. Careful studies of these residual reactions are required to determine if one of the currently understood mechanisms is responsible for these reactions, or to determine if there is yet another mechanism responsible for these events. It is also interesting to note that the apheresis platelets appear to be associated with lower frequencies of reactions than platelets prepared from PRP or buffy coats, even when the apheresis platelets contain 10^9 leukocytes per product. This observation must be interpreted with caution as comparisons of frequencies between different studies may not be valid, and the transfused apheresis products may have had a shorter duration of storage; however, the consistently low frequency of FNHTR reported to different types of apheresis platelets deserves further attention. Perhaps the process of collecting platelets using apheresis technology results in a product with a lower risk of reaction regardless of the number of contaminating leukocytes.

Clinical evidence for BRM in red cell products causing FNHTR

FNHTR to red cells are less frequent than reactions to platelets, and most of these reactions are preventable by post-storage leukoreduction [31]. Based on this observation, it is possible that most FNHTR to red cells are antibody mediated and not due to passive infusion of BRMs. This etiology is also supported by the observation that pro-inflammatory cytokines and chemokines do not accumulate to any significant level in the red cell product during the 42 day storage period [16,17]. However, there are several observations which suggest that BRM may be responsible for some red cell reactions. First, our laboratory has shown that the age of the red cell product was a predictor of a reaction [31]. This suggests that some type of BRM is accumulating in the red cell product during storage. In our study product age was a stronger predictor of a reaction for platelet than it was for red cell products. Secondly, the clinical study by Federowicz et al. [43] found that prestorage leukoreduced red cells had a 1.1% reaction rate which was 50% lower than the frequency of 2.2% observed with the post-storage leukoreduced product. Although this finding suggests that BRM that are leukocyte-derived may be the cause of some reactions, more definitive studies using rigorous methodological designs are necessary to confirm this observation. If it is shown that BRM play a role in causing red cell reactions, it will be a challenge to identify the exact substances that are responsible for these events, as the cytokines which appear to be responsible for platelet reactions are either undetectable or in very low concentrations in the red cell product.

Transfusion related acute lung injury (TRALI)

TRALI is an infrequent but life-threatening complication of blood transfusion that is characterized by acute respiratory distress, severe hypoxemia, bilateral pulmonary edema, fever and in some cases hypotension which usually occurs within one to six hours of the transfusion. Morbidity and mortality can be prevented with prompt respiratory support, and the signs and symptoms of the reaction usually resolve within 48 to 96 hours of the treatment. These reactions have been reported following the transfusion of blood products that contain plasma (red cells, platelets, plasma and cryoprecipitate) [1,47].

Most of these reactions (90%) appear to be caused by the passive transfer of leukocyte antibodies (HLA or neutrophil specific antibodies) in the donor plasma. This antigen-antibody reaction results in complement activation with C5a promoting neutrophil aggregation and sequestration in the microvascular of the lung. The release of enzymes, oxygen radicals and lipids from the neutrophils causes damage to the pulmonary vascular endothelium, with subsequent accumulation of fluid in the interstitium and alveoli resulting in respiratory distress. Although this may be the primary etiology of most reactions, in approximately 10% of patients leukocyte antibodies cannot be detected; hence, there may be other mechanisms responsible for some TRALI reactions [47,48].

It has been suggested that some cases of TRALI may result from the passive infusion of BRM in the plasma of the blood product [5,6,13]. If these BRM had the ability to prime neutrophils, it could explain the clinical characteristics of the leaky capillary syndrome. There are two BRM that have been shown to accumulate in stored blood products that have the potential to prime neutrophils.

Interleukin-8 (IL-8) is progressively generated in platelet concentrates during storage with mean levels of 11,600 pg/ml after five days [6]. Because of the high concentrations of IL-8 and its neutrophil chemotactic and activating functions, it has been postulated that passive transfer of IL-8 in platelet products may contribute to TRALI. Animal studies in rats have shown an association between intravenous infusion of IL-8 and acute lung injury; however, currently there are no human studies that support this cause-effect relationship [49,50].

The second BRM that may play a role in TRALI is a lipid compound that has the ability to priming neutrophil NADPH oxidase, possibly through the platelet activating receptor. These lipids increase in both red cell and platelet products during storage; however, their origin is unknown [5,13]. These lipids are detected in apheresis platelets containing less than 5×10^6 leukocytes suggesting that the leukocytes are not the source of lipid generation [5]. Because of their ability to prime neutrophils, it has been hypothesized that these BRM may play a role in TRALI. The only clinical evidence supporting this hypothesis is a study by Stillman et al [51] presently published only as an abstract. These investigators measured the priming activity of the blood products given to 20 transfused patients. Ten of the patients had clinical signs of pulmonary dysfunction post-transfusion and 10 patients had mild febrile reactions or urticaria (control group). The priming activity of the patient's plasma was also measured pre- and post-transfusion. The blood products given to the patients who developed pulmonary dysfunction had significantly higher levels of lipids with priming activity than the blood products transfused to the control group. These agents were also detectable in the pre-transfusion sera from all transfused patients. The lipid concentrations in the post-transfusion blood samples increased in the group of patients with pulmonary dysfunction but did not increase in the sera of patients having febrile and allergic reactions. These results are preliminary and although they support evidence for an association between lipids with neutrophil priming activity and TRALI, additional studies are needed to confirm this cause-effect relationship.

Allergic reactions

The clinical severity of allergic reactions can range from mild urticarial reactions to fulminant anaphylactic shock and death. Most urticarial reactions are mild and characterized by hives, rash and itching in the absence of fever. These reactions usually occur within an hour of initiating the transfusion and are more common when plasma products are transfused. The cause of these reactions has been attributed to an antigen-antibody reaction involving a foreign protein or substance in the transfused donor plasma that reacts with antibody in the recipient's blood, causing an immediate hypersensitivity reaction [1]. The signs and symptoms associated with this reaction are the result of histamine release by mast cells following the attachment of the allergen to IgE antibodies bound to the mast cell surface. When the response is local, the patient presents with hives. If the response is more systemic, the released histamine causes smooth muscle contraction, increased mucus secretion in the nasal and bronchial airways, and increased vascular permeability. The antigen-IgE antibody reactions are not the cause of all allergic reactions as the more severe form resulting in anaphylaxis can also be caused by an IgA antibody-antigen interaction which occurs in some IgA deficient patients [15,52].

Work by Frewin and colleagues has also suggested that some allergic reactions to blood transfusion may be caused by the passive transfer of histamine which they have shown increases in red cell products during storage [20]. They showed that virtually all the histamine present in CPDA blood and blood stored in additive solutions was released into the plasma by 42 days of storage, with mean concentrations reaching as high as 74 ng/ml. When the leukocytes were removed from the red cell products the plasma concentration of histamine after 42 days of storage was significantly decreased (mean of approximately 3 ng/ml in CPDA blood and 7 ng/ml in the blood stored in additive solutions) [53].

In a clinical study of transfusion reactions reported two years later by the same authors, it was shown that reactions to red cells that involved skin reactions tended to be associated with older red cell units [54]. The mean age of the red cell units associated with a rash was 12.4 (SD 6.9) days compared to 10.9 (SD 6.9) days for the red cell units that did not cause reactions. The investigators also found that the mean plasma histamine level measured in patients at the time that they reacted was significantly higher in the patients whose symptoms included rash, wheezing and flushing (>1 ng/ml) compared to mean levels below 0.5 ng/ml in patients who had febrile reactions or no reaction to the transfusion. It is not clear whether the increased histamine levels in the patients having allergic reactions was *in vivo* histamine generation or due in part to the passive transfer of histamine in the red cell product. Histamine levels were not measured in the blood products to determine if a correlation existed. This is currently the only clinical evidence to suggest that the passive transfusion of histamine may initiate some allergic reactions. Further studies are required to determine if this BRM in the red cell product is responsible for some of the adverse effects associated with transfusion.

Conclusion

The clinical evidence that supports a cause-effect relationship between cytokines present in platelet and red cell products and FNHTRs has been summarized. There are a number of observations suggesting that the passive infusion of BRM in platelet products are responsible for FNHTRs; however, the proof that the pro-inflammatory cytokines are the responsible agents is based only on associations and biological feasibility. It may never be possible to tease out the individual agent or agents responsible for these events because of the large number of BRM that may be generated during blood product storage and the interactions that take place. The evidence in support of this mechanism for red cell reactions is less convincing. There is preliminary clinical evidence which suggests that BRM in red cell and platelet products may contribute to TRALI and allergic reaction; however, more definitive studies are needed in these areas.

Acknowledgements

Special thanks to Janice Butera, Barbara Lahie and Luba Klama for their clerical assistance during the preparation of this manuscript.

REFERENCES

1. Heddle NM. Noninfectious adverse reactions to blood transfusion. In: Current Therapy In Haematology-Oncology. Brain MC, Carbone PP, eds, Mosby-YearBook Inc., St. Louis, MI, 1995:p225-30.

2. AABB Annual Meeting Serminar. In: Transfusion-Transmitted Viral Diseases, Moore SB (ed) American Association of Blood Banks, Arlington, VA, 1987.
3. Davenport RD, Kunkel SL. Cytokine roles in hemolytic and nonhemolytic transfusion reactions. Transf Med Rev 1994;VIII:157-68.
4. Muylle L, Joos M, Wouters E, de Bock R, Peetermans ME. Increased tumour necrosis factor α (TNFα), interleukin 1, and interleukin 6 (IL-6) levels in the plasma of stored platelet concentrates: relationship between TNFα and IL-6 levels and febrile transfusion reactions. Transfusion 1993;33:195-99.
5. Silliman C, Thurman G, Ambruso D. Agents that prime the neutrophil (PMN) oxidase develop during routine storage of platelet concentrates. Blood 1992;80:365a.
6. Stack G, Snyder EL. Cytokine generation in stored platelet concentrates. Transfusion 1994;34:20-25.
7. Aye MT, Palmer DS, Giulivi A, Hashemi S. Effect of filtration of platelet concentrates on the accumulation of cytokines and platelet release factors during storage. Transfusion 1995;35:117-24.
8. Schleuning M, Böck M, Mempel W. Complement activation during storage of single-donor platelet concentrates. Vox Sang 1994;67:144-48.
9. Heddle NM, Klama L, Singer J, et al. The role of the plasma supernatant from platelet concentrates in transfusion reactions. N Engl J Med 1994;331:625-28.
10. Muylle L, Peetermans ME. Effect of prestorage leukocyte removal on the cytokine levels in stored platelet concentrates. Vox Sang 1994;66:14-17.
11. Kluter H, Müller-Steinhardt M, Danzer S, Wilhelm D, Kirchner H. Cytokines in platelet concentrates prepared from pooled buffy coats. Vox Sang 1995;69:38-43.
12. Miletic VD, Popovic O. Complement activation in stored platelet concentrates. Transfusion 1993;33:150-54.
13. Silliman CC, Clay KL, Thurman GW, Johnson CA, Ambruso DR. Partial characterization of lipids that develop during the routine storage of blood and prime the neutrophil NADPH oxidase. J Lab Clin Med 1994;124:684-94.
14. Snyder EL. Removal of complement chemokines and other soluble biological response modifiers, by Pall bedside leukoreduction and plasma filter. Bloodlink, Pall Biomedical Products Company, Vol. 4, 1995.
15. Snyder EL, Stack G. Febrile and nonimmune transfusion reactions. In: Rossi EC, Simon TL, Moss GS, eds. Principles of transfusion medicine. Baltimore: Williams & Wilkins, 1996:641-60.
16. Decary F, Ferner P, Giavedoni L, et al. An investigation of nonhaemolytic transfusion reactions. Vox Sang 1984;46:277-85.
17. Heddle NM, Klama L, Ball S, Tan MK, Christmas T. The effect of blood product preparation on cytokine levels. Transfusion 1996;36(Suppl):15.
18. Darbonne WC, Rice GC, Mohler MA, et al. Red blood cells are a sink for interleukin 8, a leukocyte chemotaxin. J Clin Invest 1991;88: 1362-69.
19. Heddle N, Tan M, Klama L, Shroeder J. Factors affecting cytokine production in platelet concentrates. Transfusion 1994;34:67S.
20. Frewin DB, Jonsson JR, Head RJ, Russell WJ, Beal RW. Histamine levels in stored human blood. Transfusion 1984;24:502-04.
21. Sackett DL, Haynes RB, Tugwell P. Clinical Epidemiology. A Basic Science for Clinical Medicine. Boston, MA, Little, Brown, 1985.
22. Guyatt GH, Sackett DL, Cook DJ. Evidence-based medicine: User's guide to the medical literature. II. How to use an article about therapy or prevention. Part A. Are the results of the study valid? JAMA 1994;271:59-63.
23. Guyatt GH, Sackett DL, Cook DJ. Evidence-based medicine: User's guide to the medical literature. II. How to use an article about therapy or prevention. Part B. What

are the results and will they help me in caring for my patients? JAMA 1993;270: 2598-601

24. Walker RH, ed. Technical manual. 10th ed. Arlington: American Association of Blood Banks, 1990:420.
25. Payne R. The association of febrile transfusion reactions with leuko-agglutinins. Vox Sang 1957;2:233-41.
26. Payne R, Rolfs MR. Further observations on leukoagglutinin transfusion reactions. With special reference to leukoagglutinin transfusion reactions in women. Am J Med 1960;30:449-58.
27. Perkins HA, Payne R, Ferguson J, Wood M. Nonhaemolytic febrile transfusion reactions. Quantitative effects of blood components with emphasis on isoantigenic incompatibility of leukocytes. Vox Sang 1966;11:578-600.
28. Menitove JE, McElligott MC, Aster RH. Febrile transfusion reaction: what blood component should be given next? Vox Sang 1982;41:318-21.
29. Chambers LA, Kruskall MS, Pacini DG, Donovan LM. Febrile reactions after platelet transfusion: the effect of single versus multiple donors. Transfusion 1990;30:219-21.
30. Mangano MM, Chambers LA, Kruskall MS. Limited efficacy of leukopoor platelets for prevention of febrile transfusion reactions. Am J Clin Pathol 1991;95:733-38.
31. Heddle NM, Klama LN, Griffith L, Roberts R, Shukla G, Kelton JG. A prospective study to identify the risk factors associated with acute reactions to platelet and red cell transfusions. Transfusion 1993;33:794-97.
32. Muylle L, Wouters E, de Bock R, Peetermans ME. Reactions to platelet transfusion: the effect of the storage time of the concentrate. Transfus Med 1992;2:289-93.
33. Muylle L. *Ex vivo* Cytokine Production in Blood Components: Relevant or Irrelevant. Kluwer Academic Publishers: London, Vol 32, 1994.
34. Heddle NM, Kelton JG. Febrile non-haemolytic transfusion reactions. AABB Press 1996.
35. Shimizu T, Uchigiri C, Mizuno S, Kamiya T, Kokubo Y. Adsorption of anaphylatoxins and platelet-specific proteins by filtration of platelet concentrates with a polyester leukocyte reduction filter. Vox Sang 1994;66:161-65.
36. Snyder E, Napychank P, Baril L. Removal of complement component C3a and interleukin-8 from platelet concentrate by a bedside leukodepletion filter. Transfusion 1994; 34(Suppl):31S.
37. Whitebread J, Besso N, Onunka V, Brandwein H. Reduction of C3A fragment levels following leukodepletion using a Pall PXL8 filter. Transfusion 1994;84:672a.
38. Hed J, Johansson M, Lindroth M. Complement activation according to the alternate pathway by glass and plastic surfaces and its role in neutrophil adhesion. Immunology Letters 1984;8:295-99.
39. Sevast'ianov VI, Tseytlina EA. The activation of the complement system by polymer materials and their blood compatibility. J Biomed Res 1984;18:969-78.
40. Oksanen K, Ebeling F, Kekomäki R, et al. Adverse reactions to platelet transfusions are reduced by use of platelet concentrates derived from buffy coat. Vox Sang 1994;67: 356-61.
41. Anderson KC, Gorgone BC, Wahlers E, Cook J, Barrett B, Andersen J. Preparation and clinical utility of leukocyte poor apheresis platelets. Transfus Sci 1991;12:163-70.
42. Dzieczkowski JS, Barrett BB, Nester D, et al. Characterization of reactions after exclusive transfusion of white cell-reduced cellular blood components. Transfusion 1995;35: 20-5.
43. Federowicz I, Barrett BB, Andersen JW, Urashima M, Popovsky MA, Anderson KC. Characterization of reactions after transfusion of cellular blood components that are white cell reduced before storage. Transfusion 1996;36:21-28.

44. Muir JC, Jacobson S, Herschel L, AuBuchon JP. Does pre-storage leukocyte reduction of blood components reduce the risk of febrile reactions in sensitized patients? Blood 1994;84(Suppl):1842.
45. Muir JC, Herschel L, Pickard C, auBuchon JP. Pre-storage leukocyte reduction decreases the risk of febrile reactions in sensitized platelet recipients. Transfusion 1995; 35(Suppl):45S.
46. Sacher RA. High circulating interleukin 6 levels associated with acute transfusion reaction: cause or effect? Transfusion 1993;33:962(letter).
47. Popovsky MA, Chaplin HC Jr, Moore SB. Transfusion-related acute lung injury: a neglected, serious complication of haemotherapy. Transfusion 1992;32:589-92.
48. Popovsky MA, Moore SB. Diagnostic and pathogenetic considerations in transfusion-related acute lung injury. Transfusion 1985;25:573-77.
49. Rot A. Some aspects of NAP-1 pathophysiology: lung damage caused by a blood-borne cytokine. Adv Exp Med Biol 1991;305:127-35.
50. Kunkel SL, Standiford T, Kasahara K, Strieter RM. Interleukin-8 (IL-8): the major neutrophil chemotactic factor in the lung. Exp Lung Res 1991;17:17-23.
51. Silliman C, Pitman J, Thurman G, Ambruso D. Neutrophil (PMN) priming agents develop in patients with transfusion related acute lung injury. Blood (Suppl.) 1992; 261a.
52. Jeter EK, Spivey MA. Noninfectious complications of blood transfusion. Haematology/ Oncology Clinics of North American 1995;9:187-204.
53. Frewin DB, Jonsson JR, Davis KG, et al. Effect of microfiltration on the histamine levels in stored human blood. Vox Sang 1987; 52:191-94.
54. Frewin DB, Jonsson JR, Frewin CR, et al. Influence of blood storage time and plasma histamine levels on the pattern of transfusion reactions. Vox Sang 1989;56:243-56.

ABLATIVE CHEMOTHERAPY IN SOLID TUMOUR ONCOLOGY, TECHNOLOGY IN SEARCH OF AN APPLICATION?

N.H. Mulder, P.O.M. Mulder

Introduction

Fifteen years ago, the mortality rate of ablative chemotherapy, at that time with bone marrow transplantation, was approximately 20%, despite a rigorous selection of the younger and healthier patients among those with incurable solid tumours. Major complications that led to death usually resulted from septicemic fever which was a common complication. Presently in experienced centres, mortality is usually reported to be approximately one percent. In a recent survey in North America overall mortality in the mid-nineties still was given as 5%. Although difference therefore may exist between centres and various regimens, a real improvement in safety of the procedure seems to have been achieved. This has occurred despite the fact that the upper age limit for ablative chemotherapy that is reported in series in the literature steadily rises. The vast majority of courses of ablative chemotherapy nowadays follow an uneventful pattern. There is most certainly a learning curve that has influenced these results, but of far greater importance is the application first of cytokines, later followed by the use of peripheral stem cell transplantation to overcome the period of aplasia. As it is primarily the duration of the aplastic period that determines the risk of complications, the shortening of this period by these techniques has had a major influence. These developments are not in an end stage, the most promising new addition in this field is the use of thrombocyte cytokines. Further away are protecting agents and manipulations that would limit mucositis and induce bone marrow resistance for cytotoxic drugs, by for instance gene transfer for the MDR-1 gene. Alternative sources of stem cells from foetal tissue, and improved culture techniques for stem cells open wider perspectives for application of ablative chemotherapy in solid and other tumours and also for stem cell transplantation for nonmalignant diseases. So the technological revolution moves rapidly, but the core of the problem, the limited potential of our interventions has almost been at a standstill. In solid tumours, three area's have received meaningful attention over the past decades. The vast majority of patients treated now, have breast cancer, while ovarian cancer and testicular cancer comprise small numbers of patients [1]. Two decades ago small cell lung cancer has also been a shortlived focus of attention. In the same American survey breast cancer now is the indication in 40% of all transplants, immediately followed by Non Hodgkin's lymphoma.

The concept of ablative chemotherapy is applied in all of these tumour types, without much difference in the regimens used. The relation between dose of chemotherapy and treatment-result exists for doses below the optimum for all tumour types, the advocates of high dose chemotherapy consider it likely that this relation can be extended to dose levels 5, 10 or more times the normal dose.

Ovarian cancer

Advanced ovarian cancer is sensitive to chemotherapy, especially to taxol, cis-platinum or one of its analogues containing combination chemotherapy, but the majority of patients so treated will relapse or have signs of incomplete remission after the end of the first line of treatment. Presently, no standard therapy, surgery, radio-, chemo- or immune therapy or combination of these modalities, offers a perspective for cure in that situation. However, from many of the chemotherapeutic agents active in ovarian cancer a steep dose response curve has been established and also clinical information suggests a relation between dose intensity and treatment result [2]. In a number of phase I and II studies on autologous bone marrow transplantation (ABMT), we have entered patients with ovarian cancer considered to be incurable with other treatment options [3]. In a follow up on these studies we report here the results of this form of intensive chemotherapy in 18 patients after a median observation time of the four long term survivors of more than 6 years. Patients were eligible after having received at least one previous line of chemotherapy without durable (>1 year) complete clinical, or if a second look laparotomy after induction therapy had been scheduled, pathological remission.

Eleven patients received a cyclophosphamide etoposide regimen. Seven patients received a mitoxantrone based combination. Cyclophosphamide was given in a total dose of 7 g/m^2 divided over three days, mesna was given in a dose of 4 g/m^2. Etoposide was also given over three consecutive days in a total dose of 1 g/m^2. Mitoxantrone was given in a dose of 30-60 mg/m^2 divided over 3 days, melphalan 180 mg/m^2, or cyclophosphamide 7 g/m^2 were given on the same days. Cyclophosphamide was combined with mesna.

Median age of the eighteen patients was 46 years, range 29-57. One patient had previous monochemotherapy with melphalan, all others had combination chemotherapy, 3 carboplatin based, the others cis-platinum based. Before ablative chemotherapy 9 patients had lesions less than 2 centimetres, of these 3 had microscopic evidence of residual tumour only. The others had bulky residual disease. After ablative chemotherapy there were 10 complete remissions, 9 of these were confirmed with biopsies at relaparotomy or laparoscopy. Four patients had progressive disease after recovery from the regimen, three had stable disease.

From the 10 responding patients 5 relapsed within one year, a sixth relapsed after 19 months, the 4 remaining patients are symptom free after more than 7 years. The relation between tumour bulk, response and survival is given in table 1. In this group of 18 patients there was one toxic death due to pulmonary aspergillosis. One patient required cardiopulmonary resuscitation after bone marrow reinfusion, but made an uneventful recovery. All patients had periods of fever requiring antibiotic

Table 1.

Residual disease	Number	pCR	cCR	Med. survival	> 5 yr survival
> 2 cm	4	0	0	3	0
< 2cm	14	9	10	24	4

treatment. Three patients had mucositis grade 3. The four long term disease free surviving patients had a normal life, that does not seem to be compromised by the high dose chemotherapy regimen.

Although the number of patients in this study is limited, the results permit some conclusions. The application of a high dose regimen in patients with bulky, that is more than 2 cm rest lesions, does not seem to be of value. This conclusion is in agreement with results in a much larger group of patients treated by French investigators reviewed recently [4]. Sixty-five patients with macroscopic rest lesions after various forms of induction therapy relapsed after high dose chemotherapy in subsequent years. The same analysis showed better results in a more favourable subset of patients, as in a group of 52 patients with microscopic disease after induction the 5 year progression free survival is reported to be 30%. In our group of 10 patients with low volume residual disease the 6-12 year survival is 40%. The perspective of this form of aggressive chemotherapy is therefore limited to patients who before ablative chemotherapy have only microscopic disease or at least disease confined to small nodules (<2 cm). Although these patients with conventional therapy have 5 year disease free survival comparable to those in complete remission, ultimately all of them will relapse [5].

The long term observations in our and the French studies therefore leave the possibility that ablative treatment could have value in this group of patients, at the prise of considerable toxicity as witnessed by the toxic death rates of approximately 5% in both studies.

Breast cancer

Breast cancer has become worldwide a favourite area of clinical research for this mode of treatment. The reason for this is that in a variety of stages of this disease the unfavourable prognosis can be predicted while important medical problems are still absent. Patients with disseminated disease, or inflammatory breast cancer will rarely survive with conventional chemotherapy even if a complete response is obtained. This is also true for patients with 10 or more involved axillary nodes and for almost all women with more than 5 nodes.

We have applied this high dose chemotherapy in a number of phase I, II and III studies in various stages of breast cancer over more than a decade. In this period the technology of supportive care has changed considerably, and this has influenced the choice of drugs, their dose and the schedules used.

In phase I studies we have developed two groups of regimens. The first consisted of cyclophosphamide in its established dose of 7 g/m^2 (Escalation Factor 6) combined with etoposide, for which we established a dose of 1.2 g/m^2 (E.F. 4). At this and higher dose levels etoposide was found to be active in breast cancer. The second group of regimens was based on mitoxantrone [6] at a dose of 60 mg/m^2 (E.F. 4). This drug could be combined with melphalan 180 mg/m^2 or thiotepa 800 mg/m^2 (E.F. 16). This last drug remains by far the one that can be escalated to the highest level with relatively minor toxicity consisting of mucositis, controllable with cooling of the mouth with ice, and limited hepatotoxicity.

We have most recently given thiotepa as a first ablative course followed by melphalan/mitoxantrone after recovery from extramedullary toxicity. In this setting this first treatment part can be given on an outpatient base.

Patients with metastatic disease responding to first line chemotherapy were treated in phase I studies and in phase II studies aimed at determining the scope of the cyclophosphamide-etoposide regimen. Out of 13 patients treated, two remain free of disease after more than 6 years, both patients had initially presented with extensive lung, liver and bone metastases. The other 11 patients all died from disease progression within 18 months after intensive chemotherapy. The median survival was clearly not influenced in this small study. However, the occurrence of long-term disease free survival in small numbers of patients was considered to be stimulating.

Therefore, the Dutch working group on ABMT in solid tumours adapted the mitoxantrone-melphalan regimen in a phase II study in patients who were in complete remission from first line chemotherapy for metastatic breast cancer. In this multicentre study 30 patients were entered with a median age of 42. There was one toxic death, mucositis was the main extramedullary toxicity. At three years the disease free survival was 43%.

The impression of these results is that long term disease free survival is relatively common in this cohort. However, recent reports have established that between 15 and 20% of patients who reach a complete remission on standard induction therapy will have prolonged disease free survival without any further treatment.

To further analyze the possible advantage of ablative chemotherapy in metastatic breast cancer we initiated a randomized study. Today 30 patients have been treated with a tandem of thiotepa followed by melphalan and mitoxantrone or no further therapy after induction. The control group has a 15% disease free survival, the treatment group 40% at three years. This study will be continued.

An interesting study used the cyclophosphamide-etoposide regimen (10 patients) or the mitoxantrone-thiotepa regimen (30 patients) in women with 5 or more positive axillary nodes. All of these patients received the same induction treatment and radiotherapy was given in case of extranodal tumour. All patients received tamoxifen for two years after treatment. Median age of these patients was 42, the median number of lymph nodes involved was 10. In this group there was one toxic death and one death during follow up, possibly related to treatment (cardiac death). Radiation pneumonitis occurred in 50% of patients. Two relapses occurred in the brain. At a median observation of 6 years, disease free survival is 72%, 10 year disease free survival is 66%.

This study is now followed by a randomized study in a comparable group of patients, performed by the Dutch working group on ABMT. This study has now entered more than 400 patients.

Although the concept of high dose chemotherapy for solid tumours, and particularly breast cancer, has been applied for more than a decade, an explosive increase in the numbers of patients treated this way has followed the development of growth factor technology and peripheral stem cell transfusion. Despite this immense activity the role for this form of treatment in such a common malignancy as breast cancer remains unresolved.

The literature on this subject shows in phase II studies essentially the same results that our study gave: disease free survival up to twice the percentage for conservative treatment in patients with a high nodal state [7].

In metastatic breast cancer two phase III studies have been reported. A South African group found superior survival for the ablative group [8], although even in that group only 20% long term survivors were reported. In an American study from the group of Peters, not yet reported in full, a modest increase in remission duration was found in the group with ablative chemotherapy. The control group received this ablative treatment on relapse and this sequence scored the longest survival. This finding does not seem to fit the perspective of cure in metastatic breastcancer.

Salvage therapy for testicular cancer

Although testicular cancer is exquisitely sensitive for chemotherapy, in particular for cisplatin, cure remains elusive for approximately 20% of patients. Unfavourable characteristics at presentation, such as extremely high tumour markers, large numbers of metastatic sites especially in parenchymatous organs are thought to reflect the risk of treatment failure.

As cisplatinum is the cornerstone of chemotherapy, resistance of the tumour to this drug manifest during treatment is a grave sign and so is the occurrence of relapse early after seemingly successful induction.

In all of these three situations the risk of death from tumour progression is high enough to consider an alternative to standard therapy. At present there is no alternative to chemotherapy in metastatic germ cell cancer. Neither immunotherapy or other biological response modifiers nor hormonal approaches are promising.

It is also unlikely that any existing cytotoxic drugs or combinations have been systematically overlooked. New drugs, especially with different modes of action are scarce, the latest addition to the armamentarium has been Taxol, but this has only a modest response rate in testicular cancer.

Therefore high dose chemotherapy has intensively been studied for germ cell cancer. The spectrum of drugs that have been escalated in dose in germ cell cancer is extremely small. All studies use carboplatin, nearly all etoposide, a few iphosphamide or cyclophosphamide (9,10). In most studies two ablative courses are attempted, a preceding intensive course of the same drugs is sometimes given.
The choice of carboplatin seems logical in view of the sensitivity of germ cell cancer to cisplatinum. However in *in vitro* models germ cell lines resistant to

cisplatin, usually between 2-15 times, have the same order of sensitivity as breast- or colon cancer cells. The escalation potential of carboplatin is low, maximally tolerated dose seems to be around 2000 mg/m^2, but most studies use 1600 mg/m^2 or less. The escalation factor is no more than 4, the same as for etoposide. Most alkylators permit higher escalations. Alternatives for carboplatin have not emerged. In the clinical testing of platinum analogues it should be kept in mind that provided dose escalation is possible there may be a place for a drug that has no superior activity or toxicity profile.

The number of courses may also be critical, even the most sensitive tumour will not be cured by one single course. Assuming an increase in resistance that is barely less than the dose increment it is naive to expect cure from a single dose of ablative therapy.

Which testicular cancer patients can be considered for ablative therapy?

(1) Patients at high risk for failure of first line treatment: To determine if a patient is at sufficient risk to allow experimental therapy in first line a classification system that has prospectively been tested should assign such a patient a small chance of cure, probably no more than 10 or 20%, with conventional therapy.

A study that randomizes patients with those characteristics to some form of ablative therapy, with repeated courses, or conservative treatment can answer the question of the place of upfront intensive therapy. Studies aspiring this goal are in progress in Europe.

(2) Patients relapsing after conservative treatment: Patients relapsing after induction treatment are defined as having experienced a clinical, biochemical remission after platinum containing treatment. After at least 4 weeks since last treatment tumour activity becomes evident. Pathological conformation is usually required to exclude mature teratoma.

This is a heterogeneous group of patients. At one end of the spectrum is the rare patient relapsing 2 years after etoposide and cisplatin. Such a patient can be cured by repeating the same treatment. At the other end are patients with high volume disease who relapse 3 months after an intensified regimen with both cisplatin and iphosphamide. These patients have a small chance for cure with a repeated regimen. Probably patients who relapse within a year after a first or later line containing these two drugs should be considered candidates for high dose regimens.

From the literature we have assembled a group of 48 patients who seem to fit these criteria. In this group there were 9 long term disease free survivors, long term defined as close to or more than a year, this probably means cure for this tumour.

(3) Patients resistant to cisplatin: Patients who have not acquired a complete response on platinum containing treatment, or who relapse within a month, who can not be rendered disease free by surgery, have a grave prognosis.

This is true irrespective whether first or another line of treatment is concerned. In the literature 72 patients were reported with 13 long term disease free survivors, also 18%.

The total number of patients dying during ablative treatment is 14 of 120 or 12%.

The total number of patients dying during ablative treatment is 14 of 120 or 12%.

In some of the studies subgroups are described who can not be cured, such as patients relapsing or refractory with extragonadal tumours, or patients without any response to previous cisplatin.

How should these results be interpreted?

Clearly the prospects for patients entered in these regimens are grim, the chance of being cured is not much higher than the chance of being killed. However they offer a chance, and probably more experience with stem cell infusion and growth factors will lead to smaller numbers of toxic deaths.

Can we recommend a particular ablative regimen currently in use for these three groups although some results seem to be better than other reports, usually the regimens are comparable, indicating that the difference is mainly due to patient selection.

Would it be informative to perform a randomised study?

There is no control treatment available: an iphosphamide cisplatin combination repetition after previous failure is even more unattractive than no treatment. Other ways of modulating cisplatin resistance could be considered, for instance the use of BSO in order to decrease tumour gluthation levels, in combination with carboplatin in a nonablative dose.

It might be worthwhile to reconsider other drugs that can be given in such regimens; thiotepa, with an escalation factor of more than 100, melphalan 7, high dose methotrexate. To test these approaches in randomised phase II or III studies against a "standard" ablative regimen seems defendable in view of the limited scope of these ablative regimens.

Conclusion

The results of our group and others in the treatment of solid tumours, reviewed above, show that ablative chemotherapy has become a common treatment modality also in solid tumours. The technology of supporting and salvaging bone marrow function has grown impressively over the last years. As yet the therapeutic effects are limited: it is a reasonable option in selected germ cell cancers. There is considerable hope that an indication will emerge in the adjuvant setting in breast cancer. The place in metastatic breast cancer is experimental, in all other tumours the evidence is against ablative chemotherapy.

References

1. Antman KH, Souhami RL. High-dose chemotherapy in solid tumours. Ann Onc 1993;4 (Suppl 1):29-44.
2. Kaye SB, Paul J, Cassidy J, et al. Mature results of a randomized trial of two doses of cisplatin for the treatment of ovarian cancer. J Clin Oncol 1996;14:2113-19.

3. Mulder POM, Willemse PHB, Aalders JG, et al. High-dose chemotherapy with autologous bone marrow transplantation in patients with refractory ovarian cancer. Eur J Cancer Clin Oncol 1989;25:645-49.
4. De Vries EGE, Hamilton TC, Lind M, Dauplat J, Neijt JP, Ozols RF. Drug resistance, supportive care and dose intensity. Ann Oncol 1993;4(Suppl 4):57-62.
5. Neijt JP, Ten Bokkel Huinink WW, Van der Burg MEL, et al. Long-term survival in ovarian cancer. Eur J Cancer 1991;27:1367-72.
6. Mulder POM, Sleijfer DTh, Willemse PHB, de Vries EGE, Uges DRA, Mulder NH. High-dose cyclophosphamide or melphalan with escalating doses of mitoxantrone and autologous bone marrow transplantation for refractory solid tumours. Cancer Res 1989;49:4654-58.
7. Peters WP, Ross M, Vredenburgh JJ, et al. High-dose chemotherapy and autologous bone marrow support as consolidation after standard-dose adjuvant therapy for high-risk primary breast cancer. J Clin Oncol 1993;11:1132-43.
8. Bezwoda WR, Seymour L, Dansey RD. High-dose chemotherapy with haematopoietic rescue as primary treatment for metastatic breast cancer: A randomized trial. J Clin Oncol 1995;13:2483-2489.
9. Mulder POM, de Vries EGE, Schraffordt Koops H, et al. Chemotherapy with maximally tolerable doses of VP 16-213 and cyclophosphamide followed by autologous bone marrow transplantation for the treatment of relapsed or refractory germ cell tumours. Eur J Cancer Clin Oncol 1988;24:675-79.
10. Barnett MJ, Coppin CML, Murray N, et al. High-dose chemotherapy and autologous bone marrow transplantation for patients with poor prognosis nonseminomatous germ cell tumours. Br J Cancer 1993;68:594-98.

GENE THERAPY IN MALIGNANCIES: DEVELOPMENT AND CLINICAL APPLICATIONS OF AUTOLOGOUS TUMOUR VACCINES

J.I. Drayer

Introduction

Various applications of therapeutically active cancer vaccines have recently been reviewed by Subiza et al. [1]. In their opinion, concepts and tools related to such therapies are more clear than ever before and clinical results are encouraging. Accompanying editorials express somewhat contrasting views. In one editorial the need is expressed for a combination of antigen-specific effect targeting the immune reaction to tumour plus a systemic immuno- or endocrine-modulating effect to treat cancer [2], and in the potential of the other producing progression or only temporary benefit following vaccine therapy [3].

In this article, preliminary results will be presented from clinical trials using a genetically modified autologous tumour cell vaccine (GVAX™ Cancer Vaccine), in patients with renal cell carcinoma and melanoma. The local and systemic immune response to vaccinations will be described including its effect on residual or recurrent disease.

GVAX™ cancer vaccine

The GVAX™ Cancer Vaccine (GVAX) is an irradiated autologous human tumour cell vaccine that consists of cultured tumour cells genetically modified with a retroviral vector encoding the human cytokine GM-CSF. The clinical development of GVAX is based upon a series of preclinical murine tumour model studies. In these experiments, the development of anti-tumour immunity was evaluated following vaccination with a murine melanoma cell line modified to express different cytokines and cell surface proteins [4]. The cytokine GM-CSF was shown to be more potent than others in protection from subsequent potentially lethal challenge with live tumour cells. In addition, animals with pre-existing tumours were shown to have a complete response following vaccinations. Multiple tumour types have been tested, revealing similar results. The immunity obtained was tumour specific and required both CD8 and CD4 positive lymphocytes. The pathology of the vaccine site revealed infiltrates of granulocytes, eosinophils, lymphocytes, as well as dendritic cells. Preclinical pharmacokinetic experiments have shown a minimal effective cell dose of 5×10^5 cells/vaccination and a minimally effective dose of GM-CSF (approximately 40 ng/10^6 cells/24 hours) are required to induce the desired anti-tumour response (Somatix' Investigator's Brochure).

Clinical trial in renal cell carcinoma

In a phase I clinical trial, patients with stage IV (metastatic) renal cell carcinoma were randomly assigned to receive equivalent GM-CSF transduced or non-transduced cell doses of GVAX™ at 3 escalating dose levels [5].

Up to 4 vaccinations of 4×10^6, 4×10^7 or 4×10^8 cells per vaccine were given at 4 week intervals at each dose level. GM-CSF secretion was less than 40 ng/10^6 cells/24 hours in all patients in the non-transduced group and greater than 40 ng/10^6 cells/24 hours in all but one patient in the transduced group. A total of 18 patients were treated (10 non-transduced and 8 transduced) and these patients received a total of 44 vaccinations.

No dose limiting toxicities were encountered and transduced vaccines produced no greater toxicities than non-transduced vaccines.

The DTH response to autologous non-transduced tumour cells was cell dose dependent and greater in patients receiving the transduced vaccine. The largest DTH response was seen in one patient who had a partial clinical response to therapy. Analyses of biopsies at the vaccine and DTH sites showed cellular infiltrates that were qualitatively similar to those observed in preclinical models and included granulocytes, lymphocytes and eosinophils [6,7].

Clinical trials in melanoma

Preliminary data from two ongoing studies will be reported. In a phase I study cell doses of 5×10^6 or 5×10^7 per vaccination were given for 3 vaccinations at 3 week intervals in patients with stage IV (metastatic) melanoma. Fourteen patients will be treated at each of these dose levels. As of June 1996, twenty-one patients have completed the trial, 14 at the low cell dose and 7 at the high dose. GM-CSF secretion rates were greater than 40 ng/10^6 cells/24 hours in all patients (range 95 to 980 ng/10^6 cells/24 hours).

Toxicities consisted of erythaema, induration and pruritis at the injection site and were more intense after multiple vaccinations and at the higher dose level. Biopsies from vaccine and DTH sites showed increased number of Langerhans cells, lymphocytes, including perivascular CD4 positive lymphocytic infiltration, and eosinophils. An increase in eosinophils in peripheral blood was noted following vaccinations. Increases in precursor cytotoxic T cells have been seen in several patients. Changes in distant residual metastases include erythaema, lymphocytic infiltration and regression of subcutaneous lesions. Lymphocytic infiltrates were seen in selected lesions studied. Protracted stabilization (>6 months) of previously progressive disease was noted [8].

In a second study, vaccinations of 10^7 cells were administered at time intervals of four, two and one week for 3 months (3, 6 and 12 vaccinations respectively) in patients with stage IV (metastatic) melanoma [9].

As of June 1996, three patients received 3 vaccinations at intervals of 4 weeks, four received 6 vaccinations at intervals of 2 weeks, and three received 12 vaccinations at intervals of 1 week. Ten additional patients will be given 12 vaccinations at intervals of 1 week. GM-CSF secretion rates ranged from 136 to 583 ng/10^6 cells/24 hours.

Local reactions at the vaccine sites included erythaema, induration and pruritis, most often after multiple vaccinations and when the vaccinations were given at shorter intervals. Significant increases in eosinophil counts in peripheral blood were seen.

Biopsies of vaccination and DTH sites revealed marked infiltrates of lymphocytes, dendritic cells, macrophages and eosinophils. DTH reactions also were characterized by dense infiltrates of lymphocytes, macrophages and eosinophils. Pathologic analyses of sites of distant residual tumour demonstrated similar infiltrates. In these lesions evidence of direct toxic effects on tumour cells were seen with various degrees of apoptosis and necrosis of tumour cells. Dense fibrosis with areas of lymphocytic and eosinophil infiltrates also were seen at these metastatic sites.

Safety of GVAX™

In total, including all ongoing studies with GVAX, more than 250 vaccinations have been given to more than 70 patients with various types of metastatic cancer. Follow-up has extended beyond 24 months in some patients. The safety profile of GVAX has been remarkable, with only few reported serious adverse events that were considered possibly related to GVAX. These events were resolved with minimal medical intervention. Non-serious adverse events were mostly local reactions at the vaccination site and these tended to increase with cell dose, with the number of vaccinations and with decreased intervals between vaccinations.

All patients were tested repeatedly for replication competent retroviral events (RCR), but non were detected. Signs, symptoms or laboratory test results indicative of any form of autoimmune disease have not been observed.

Discussion

Preliminary data are presented from studies designed to induce active immunotherapy by administration of autologous tumour cells that have been altered genetically to secrete the cytokine GM-CSF. This form of active immunotherapy was chosen over other types of immunotherapy because of the marked results seen in preclinical studies. The results from clinical data in early clinical trials have been most encouraging.

Since safety is a primary endpoint in early clinical trials, it is important to note that, at least for a period of up to 24 months, no events have been observed that caused reason to discontinue therapy. The few serious adverse events seen were treated using short-term supportive medication (e.g.: antihistamines). Other adverse events were mostly confined to local reactions at the site of vaccination. The nature of the safety profile is such that this form of therapy can be given on an outpatient basis and that most patients will not need to interfere significantly with their normal activities. Obviously, this daily profile is vastly different from that of other cancer therapies, such as radiation and chemotherapy.

In these studies, a number of patients were not able to receive the full course of therapy defined in the protocol. In almost all cases, this was due to progression of disease and/or lack of response to conventional therapy given during the period of time needed to produce and test the vaccine. As anticipated, the local immune response to vaccinations was less in patients who received fewer vaccines and in those with a large and progressively growing tumour burden prior to the start of vaccinations. Poor clinical outcome was observed in most of these patients.

The similarities in the results between those in metastatic renal cell carcinoma and metastatic melanoma was remarkable. The safety profile was comparable and related to cell dose, GM-CSF secretion rate and the number of vaccinations given. In addition, local signs of immune response measured by the responses seen at vaccination and DTH sites were comparable between the tumour types and dependent upon the same factors.

In both tumour types, cell doses of 1×10^7 or greater per vaccine seemed to generate more consistent and stronger responses than lower cell doses. Results from the clinical trials in stage IV melanoma further emphasized the importance of the dosing interval, with more potent responses when vaccines are given at intervals of 1 to 2 weeks than at intervals of 3 to 4 weeks. The strongest immune responses seen were observed after 3 vaccinations with 4×10^7 cells in renal cell carcinoma and after 6 or more vaccinations with 1×10^7 cells given at intervals of 1 week. Significant signs of DTH response has been seen in all patients who received 3 or more vaccinations with GM-CSF transduced autologous tumour cells.

Interestingly, other signs of immune response were seen, including increases in eosinophils in peripheral blood especially in patients with melanoma. This may be caused by a direct effect of GM-CSF or by activation of other cytokines.

Further pathological and immunohistochemistry evaluation of biopsies taken from vaccination sites, DTH sites and residual or recurrent tumour sites have provided more evidence for the induction of a significant tumour directed immune response following therapy with GVAX. It can be concluded from the data obtained in the study in renal cell carcinoma that transduction with GM-CSF is mandatory to obtain a significant immune response. Eosinophils were present only in patients treated with transduced tumour cells. Evaluation of biopsies from both patients with renal cell carcinoma and melanoma confirm similarities in the response and observations that closely match findings in preclinical models.

Marked cellular responses were seen at vaccine and DTH sites with dense infiltrates of eosinophils, T-lymphocytes and plasma cells. This confirms the presence of a multifaceted immune response involving non-specific responses, specific non-cellular responses and specific cellular immune responses. Most importantly, similar infiltrates were seen at sites of residual tumour following vaccination. Metastatic lesions examined following vaccinations have shown evidence of apoptosis and necrosis of tumour cells. In addition, such sites revealed clinical signs of inflammation and symptoms comparable to those seen at the vaccine site.

These findings have been observed in some patients who received at least 3 vaccinations, but more consistently in patients who received 6 or more vaccinations, particularly in patients with smaller and less progressive tumour burden at the time of vaccination.

Repeated DTH test following vaccination have revealed continued evidence of an immune response until at least 12 months following vaccination (personal communication by Dr. E. Rankin).

Work is ongoing on the detection of tumour specific cytotoxic T-cells in blood and residual tumour following vaccination. In a number of patients, the presence of these T-cells has been confirmed.

Based on these observations, it seems reasonable to conclude that active immunotherapy of cancer has reached the clinic and that important information has been gained on the useful dose and dosing regimen for GVAX. In addition, preclinical and clinical information, support the concept that effective tumour directed immune response resulting in tumour necrosis and a clinical partial response in at least one patient, can be obtained. Multiple parts of the immune system seem to be involved in this response.

Therefore, it might be reasonable, to be more optimistic on the potential efficacy of immune therapy of cancer using gene modified autologous tumour cell vaccines. However, additional trials in larger patient populations will need to be conducted to firmly establish the efficacy of this therapy.

Based on our findings, and on information presented in various recent review articles [10,11] a number of issues should be considered in the design of efficacy trials using active immunotherapy.

The patients selected for these trials should have a minimal tumour burden at the time of therapy. It probably is not needed to confine therapy to the adjuvant setting and patients with some residual disease and no signs of rapid progression could be included in clinical trials. This is particularly important for gene modified autologous vaccine which, at least using current technology, may require a period of 6 to 8 weeks to release. However, use of different vectors and future improvement in processes for cell growth and testing could potentially reduce this period to 2 weeks or less.

It is important to recognize differences in anti-tumour responses by chemotherapy or active immune therapy. As reported in this article and by others [12], it may take some time to reach maximum activation of the immune system and the subsequent clinical response. Because of the significant infiltrates and pathological changes (necrosis and fibrosis), induced at metastatic sites it may be less likely to demonstrate tumour shrinkage using standard radiologic procedures. In fact, survival may be a more appropriate endpoint in these trials. In the presence of significant tumour burden at the start of therapy, other therapy may need to be considered prior to, or following vaccination therapy.

In summary, active immunotherapy has passed the first hurdle of clinical development and a large number of efficacy trials using a variety of such therapies have started or will be started in the near future. From here on, it will be possible to arrive at more definitive statements on the efficacy of immunotherapy around the year 2000.

References

1. Subiza JL, Cifuentes L, Medina MT. Prospects in cancer vaccines. Cancer J 1995; 8:293-98.
2. Fridman WH. Cancer vaccines – Myth or reality? Cancer J 1995;8:188-90.
3. Prehn RT. On the probability of effective anticancer vaccines. Cancer J 1995;8:284-85.
4. Dranoff G, Jaffee E, Lazenby A, et al. Vaccination with irradiated tumor cells engineered to secrete murine granulocyte-macrophage colony-stimulating factor stimulates potent, specific, and long-lasting antitumor immunity. Proc Natl Acad Sci 1993;90: 3539-43.
5. Berns A, Cohen L, Donehower RC. Phase I study of non-replicating autologous tumor cell injections using cells prepared with or without GM-CSF gene transduction in patients with renal cell carcinoma. Hum Gene Ther 1996;6:347-68.
6. Simons J, Jaffee EM, Weber C, et al. Bioactivity of human GM-CSF gene transfer in autologous irradiated renal cell carcinoma vaccines. J Clin Oncol 1997 (in press).
7. Pardoll DM. GM-CSF transfected autologous RC vaccine. Presented at the NCI-EORTC Conference, March 1996, Amsterdam, The Netherlands.
8. Rankin E. Immunological effects of vaccination with autologous, GM-CSF transduced and irradiated tumor cells in patients with advanced melanoma. Presented at the NCI-EORTC Conference, March 1996, Amsterdam, The Netherlands.
9. Dranoff G. Granulocyte-macrophage colony stimulating factor based melanoma vaccines. Presented at the Molecular Medicine Society Conference, May 1996, Washington DC.
10. Morton DL, Barth A. Vaccine therapy for malignanat melanoma. CA Cancer J Clin 1996;46:225-44.
11. Baltz JK. Vaccines in the treatment of cancer. Am J Health Syst Pharm 1995;52: 2574-85.

VACCINATION STRATEGIES TO INDUCE T-CELL IMMUNITY AGAINST TUMOURS

M.E. Ressing, R.E.M. Toes, R.M.P. Brandt, E.I.H. van der Voort, J.H. de Jong, W.M. Kast[1], R. Offringa, C.J.M. Melief

Introduction

Effector T cells recognize immunogenic peptides that are presented on the cell membrane in the context of major histocompatibility complex (MHC) molecules. The vast majority of T cells consists of either CD8+ cytotoxic T lymphocytes (CTL) or CD4+ T helper cells. By and large, MHC class I molecules present antigenic peptides to CTL, whereas T helper cells recognize antigenic peptides in the context of MHC class II molecules. These proteins are mainly found on the cells of the immune system with a specialized antigen presenting function. In general, CD4+ lymphocytes secrete cytokines upon triggering that controles the activation of B cells, macrophages and CD8+ cells. MHC class I molecules are expressed on the cell surface of virtually all nucleated cells and present peptides derived from endogenously synthesized proteins to CTL. This enables the CTL to screen almost all cells of the body for antigenic peptides that may be presented as a consequence of viral infection or malignant transformation. Therefore, the CD8+ CTL represent a major effector subset of tumour-specific T cells responsible for rejection of tumours.

The specificity and power of the T cell section of the cellular arm of the immune system may provide new therapeutic approaches for cancer, as an extension, or even, in certain cases, replacement, of conventional cancer treatment consisting of surgery, radiotherapy and chemotherapy. Conventional cancer treatment has made modest progress in recent years, despite much effort. For cervical carcinoma – still an important cause of cancer-related death, predominantly in developing countries – no major decrease in mortality from the disease has been achieved since 1950 [1]. Moreover, the side effects of radio- and chemotherapy on healthy tissues constitute a severe complication of these types of cancer treatment. For these reasons, immunotherapy of cancer aiming at increasing the power and redirecting the specificity of the patients' immune system to attack malignant cells is now emerging.

1. Cancer Immunology Program, Loyola University Cancer Center, 2160 South First Ave., Maywood, IL 60153, USA.

Tumour antigens

Tumour-associated antigens recognized by T cells can be derived either from viral proteins, when the tumour has a viral etiology, or can be encoded by normal or mutated cellular genes [2-7].

Viral tumour antigens

Viral proteins in virus-induced tumours are ideal target structures for tumour-reactive T cells because they are tumour-specific. Especially immunogenic peptides recognized by T cells originating from viral (onco)proteins involved in transformation represent attractive immunotherapeutic targets, as evasion of immune recognition through loss of oncoprotein expression would also entail loss of the transformed state. Approximately 15% of all human tumours are virus-associated [reviewed in 8,9]. For instance, human papillomavirus (HPV) DNA can be detected in more than 90% of cervical carcinomas, predominantly of the HPV 16 and HPV 18 genotypes. These types of HPV, as well as other high-risk HPVs, have been implicated in the etiology of cervical cancer [10]. In the majority of cervical tumour cells, early regions 6 and 7 (E6 and E7) are constitutively expressed and are required for maintenance of the transformed state [11,12]. Consequently, these proteins receive most of the attention in the development of vaccination strategies against cervical cancer [13].

Cellular tumour antigens

Malignant transformation is the end result of altered expression of genes that play a pivotal role in the regulation of normal cell growth control and differentiation. This altered expression can result from gene amplification, somatic mutation, or gene translocation, yielding proteins that potentially serve as tumour-associated antigens. In mice, elegant pioneer experiments by Boon and co-workers resulted in the identification of a tumour-associated antigen recognized by CTL on the chemically modified P815 mastocytoma [14]. This gene (called P1A) is specifically expressed in the tumour cells, and has little or no expression in normal cells, explaining the antigenicity of P1A. However, T cell epitopes derived from more ubiquitously expressed tumour-associated antigens such as ras and p53 have also been identified [15-17; Vierboom, et al. unpublished observations]. Among the T cell-mediated anti-tumour responses presently characterized in cancer patients, CTL directed against cellular proteins that are encoded by mutated (onco)genes; ectopically expressed, non-mutated antigens (such as members from the MAGE-family), or lineage-specific antigens including tyrosinase, gp100, and CEA are identified [reviewed in 4,18]. From this still increasing number of identified tumour antigens, those that are specific for transformed cells, preferably involved in maintaining the malignant state and shared by multiple (types of) cancers, constitute the most attractive targets for immunotherapy in the clinic.

Indications for anti-tumour immunity

The identification of tumour-associated antigens and antigenic peptides has firmly established the existence of tumour-associated T cell targets both in murine tumour-models and in cancer patients. The notion that T cells can potentiate anti- tumour responses came from animal tumour models, in which adoptive transfer of tumour-specific T cells resulted in eradication of established tumours [reviewed in 5,19,20]. But also, in the human situation it has been reported that CTL can exert anti-tumour activity. For example, *ex vivo* expanded autologous tumour-infiltrating lymphocytes displayed therapeutic activity in patients with malignant melanoma [21].

For most human tumours (e.g. cervical carcinoma), involvement of T cell-mediated immunity in control of the disease is based on circumstantial evidence. An increased prevalence of HPV-associated proliferative disorders in immuno-suppressed patients indicates that progression of HPV infection is affected by the cellular arm of the immune response [22]. Also reports on associations of certain HLA types in the affected population with HPV-related dysplasia support a role for HPV-directed T cells [23-27]. Likewise, cervical carcinoma cells appear to have developed mechanisms to escape from CTL-mediated immune-attack by down-regulation of HLA class I expression, suggesting a role of CTL in anti-tumour surveillance [28-30]. Furthermore, clinical regression of cervical lesions has been described after biopsy [31,32]. This phenomenon may be mediated by T cells that are activated by antigen presenting cells (APC) attracted to the site of tissue disruption.

Nonetheless, despite the presence of (several) tumour-associated antigens, and the indications that T cells play a pivotal role in anti-tumour-surveillance, tumours have developed even in patients that display no overt immunodeficiency. This indicates that the immune system is not always effective, strongly encouraging the development of immune-intervention strategies. For the development of optimal T cell-based anti-cancer intervention protocols, it is necessary to conduct studies disclosing the various features of the immune system, both in a clinical setting as well as in pre-clinical animal models. The latter can be used as a guide for the clinical development of immunotherapy for cancer patients.

Murine tumour models

Protective immune responses induced by peptide-based vaccines

Because MHC class I presented peptides are the key elements recognized by CTL, vaccination with tumour-derived synthetic peptides, recognized by tumour-specific CTL, should adequately activate the hosts immune system. Indeed, sub-cutaneous vaccination of mice with a peptide representing a T cell epitope emulsified in incomplete Freunds adjuvant (IFA) can induce protective immunity against viral infections and tumours as shown in several models [17,33-39].

The first tumour model in which peptide-based immune intervention led to complete tumour protection involved an HPV 16 E7-encoded CTL epitope (amino acids 49-57) presented by the murine class I H-2D^b molecule [40, 41]. Vaccination with this peptide in incomplete Freunds adjuvant (IFA) protected mice against an otherwise lethal challenge with HPV 16 transformed syngeneic tumour cells. Accordingly, CTL induced by this immunization protocol were capable of lysing peptide-pulsed target cells as well as tumour cells *in vitro*, showing the potency of peptide-based vaccines to evoke protective anti-tumour immunity. In addition to the prophylactic induction of anti-tumour immunity, peptide vaccination can also result in eradication of pre-existing tumour burdens. In several different tumour models treatment of animals bearing established macroscopic tumours with dendritic cells prepulsed with the respective tumour-specific peptides resulted in sustained tumour regression and tumour-free status in the majority of treated mice [42,43]. Likewise, vaccination with a peptide derived from a mutated connexin 37 gap-junction protein present on a murine lung carcinoma prevented metastatic spread from a primary tumour that was allowed to develop for 30 days before surgical exicision. Both peptides given in IFA and peptide loaded on cells reduced metastatic growth in mice carrying pre-established metastasis [44]. This CD8+ T cell-mediated anti-tumour effect resembles a clinical setting in which surgical debulking of the tumour might be combined with immunotherapeutic clearance of remaining tumour cells. Thus, as demonstrated by these studies, vaccination with peptides can induce protective, or even therapeutic, T cell-mediated immunity.

Adverse effects of peptide vaccination

A peptide corresponding to a CTL-epitope derived from lymphocytic chorio-meningitis virus (LCMV) is capable of inducing protective anti-viral CTL responses when administered subcutaneously in IFA. The same peptide can, however, also lead to a specific down-regulation of T cell responsiveness. Intraperitoneal injections of high doses of the LCMV-peptide induced specific CTL tolerance, when given repeatedly. This mode of peptide delivery prevented the induction of diabetes by infection with LCMV in a transgenic mouse model in which LCMV glycoprotein was expressed in the β islet cells of the pancreas [45,46]. Thus, priming versus tolerization of T cells against LCMV depended on peptide dose, route and frequency of administration.

Modulation of the T cell immune response through peptide vaccination was also studied in a tumour model. Adenovirus type 5 (Ad5) E1-transformed cells present at least two CTL epitopes to the immune system, encoded by the Ad5E1A and Ad5E1B regions [47,48]. CTL clones directed against these peptide epitopes are able to eradicate established tumours in nude mice when infused into tumour-bearing animals, showing that these epitopes can mediate tumour regression. In contrast, a single subcutaneous injection of a low dose of these peptides (1-10 μg) in IFA (or CFA) into immunocompetent animals – a mode of peptide administration proven to induce protective T cell immunity in several other models – resulted in enhanced tumour outgrowth. This was associated by specific T cell unresponsiveness *in vitro* and *in vivo* to the respective epitopes, indicating that deletion of antigen-specific CTL activity explains the enhanced outgrowth of Ad5E1-expressing tumour cells [49,50].

The reasons why certain peptides induce protective T cell mediated immunity, whereas others evoke T cell tolerance, when administered at comparable concentrations via the same vaccination scheme, are intriguing. A possible explanation is that peptides eliciting protective immune responses, such as the HPV16 E749-57-encoded peptide, are retained locally, forming a gradient of antigen, whereas the Ad5E1-peptides diffuse rapidly throughout the body, instigating downregulation of the Ad5E1-specific CTL response [49, 50]. Systemic distribution might lead to massive activation of peptide-specific CTL, which, especially if associated with inappropriate costimulation, may result in clonal exhausting of these CTL.

In conclusion, a delicate balance exists between the induction or repression of protective T cell responses by peptide vaccination and care should therefore be taken with respect to the design of peptide-based vaccines for clinical application.

Finding the right formulation

An essential aspect of developing peptide-based vaccines is the identification of adjuvants or delivery systems that facilitate the generation of controlled and reliable T cell-mediated anti-tumour immune responses.

As discussed before, dendritic cells (DC) appear a promising vehicle. To circumvent the limitations of single peptide pulsing, DC can be fed with a target protein of interest to activate both class I and class II-restricted T cell responses [51-53]. When autologous tumour cells are the only known source of tumour antigens, unfractionated acid-eluted peptides from the tumour can be pulsed onto dendritic cells [54]. A matter of concern when using DC as carriers is the labor-intensive isolation of limited amounts of cells, although recent improvements of culture techniques, making use of cytokines such as GM-CSF, has greatly enhanced the yield of DC that can be isolated from a donor.

Besides vaccination with peptide-antigens or whole proteins, also various other immunization-strategies can be employed. For instance, tumours used for vaccination purposes can be rendered more immunogenic by transfection or retroviral transduction of genes encoding cytokines or co-stimulatory molecules into tumours [reviewed in 55,56]. These genetically altered tumour cells may stimulate the immune system, resulting in specific anti-tumour immunity. The mechanism by which tumour cell-based vaccines activate T cell-mediated immunity most likely involves uptake of tumour-derived antigens by host APC, as shown in several models [57,58]. This so-called cross-priming of protective CTL-responses after tumour-cell vaccination also suggested that completely allogeneic tumour cells can be used for vaccination purposes. Indeed, immunization with completely allogeneic tumour cells, expressing specific tumour-associated antigens, evokes protective syngeneic anti-tumour immunity [59]. These data indicate that MHC-matching between tumour cells used in the vaccine and the patients' MHC becomes redundant, whereas matching of tumour-associated antigens between the tumour cell vaccine and the patient becomes obligatory. The observation that completely allogeneic tumour cells can be used as an effective vehicle for the induction of anti-tumour immunity also indicates that one tumour cell vaccine, when expressing the right tumour-associated antigens, can be used for many different patients.

Other approaches that permit a wide applicability of vaccines (with respect to antigen specificity and HLA polymorphism) include recombinant DNA or viral vectors, such as recombinant adenoviruses, expressing whole tumour antigens or multiple defined T cell epitopes in a string-of-beads fashion. Especially the latter approach seems to be very promising, since the immune response can be targeted towards multiple T cell specificities via a single immunization, thereby reducing the chance of tumour cells escaping from immune attack. Finally, in cases where active vaccination for the induction of anti-tumour immunity is not feasible, adoptive transfer of tumour-specific T cells expanded *in vitro* can be considered. As shown both in Ad5E1- and HPV 16 mouse tumour models, large established tumours can be eradicated by adoptive transfer of tumour-specific CTL [47,48].

Thus, as shown by the examples described above, current and future experiments in murine models will yield crucial knowledge for the development of immunotherapy.

Extrapolation to humans: HLA-transgenic mice and *in vitro* response inductions

Since administration of antigen can either result in induction or tolerization of T cell responses, it is important to test potential immunotherapeutic protocols extensively before applying them in a clinical setting. To this extent, T cell response inductions *in vivo* in HLA transgenic mice and *in vitro* with human peripheral blood mononuclear cells (PBMC) (donor or patient-derived) are important tools. The usefulness of testing vaccines in HLA-transgenic animals depends on their ability to raise physiologically relevant information with regard to human HLA-restricted T cell responses. For instance, transgenic mouse strains have been developed that express either the entire HLA-A*0201 or a chimeric HLA-A2K^b molecule. The latter chimeric molecule consists of α-1 and α-2 domains encoded by the human HLA-A*0201 gene and an α-3 domain of the murine H-2K^b molecule that permits a natural interaction with murine CD8 molecules. Importantly, immunization of these transgenic mice with Influenza virus or a recombinant vaccinia virus expressing the hepatitis C virus envelope and core genes yielded HLA-A2-restricted murine CTL that recognized both murine and human targets expressing the viral antigen in combination with HLA-A2 [60-66]. Moreover, the epitope specificity of the responding murine CTL was virtually identical to that of human CTL from virus-infected individuals. These data indicate that, in spite of species differences, both the antigen processing and presentation pathways as well as the T cell repertoire present, will yield a similar response in both man and mice when the same MHC class I molecule is present. Moreover, these data indicate that valuable information can be obtained about the efficacy of vaccines to be used in a clinical setting by testing these vaccines in HLA-transgenic animals.

HLA-A2 transgenic mice have been used to assess the *in vivo* immunogenicity of peptides capable of binding to HLA-A2 [67-70]. Encouraged by the protective capacity of an HPV 16-encoded peptide in mice, we undertook the identification of potential human CTL epitopes encoded by HPV16 and 18. For 5 common

HLA-A alleles – together covering the HLA allele expression of a majority of the human population – candidate epitopes encoded by HPV 16 and 18 E6 and E7 capable of binding to these MHC molecules have been identified [71,72]. Of the high affinity HLA-A*0201-binding peptides, 3 E7 peptides were found to be immunogenic both *in vivo* in HLA-A2K^b transgenic mice and *in vitro* to PBMC of healthy donors [68]. Human CD8$^+$ CTL clones against these 3 peptides lysed a human HLA-A*0201$^+$, HPV16$^+$ cervical carcinoma cell line, suggesting these peptides to represent endogenously processed human CTL epitopes of HPV 16 [68]. Furthermore, indications of natural CTL responses have been obtained against one of these peptides in a minority of HLA-A2$^+$ cervical intraepithelial neoplasia and cervical cancer patients with proven HPV 16 infections [73]. Currently, we are developing a tumour model in HLA-A2K^b transgenic mice in order to directly assess the effects of various HPV 16-based vaccination strategies on the outgrowth of syngeneic HPV 16-induced tumours.

In conclusion, the use of both animal models and *in vitro* response inductions with human material led to the identification and preclinical application of tumour antigens. The next step is to exploit the knowledge of these antigens for the development of clinical vaccination strategies aiming at the induction or augmentation of protective or therapeutic T cell-mediated immunity in human beings.

Clinical trials

The effectiveness of peptide vaccination for humans was first demonstrated in healthy volunteers, with no signs of preceeding hepatitis B virus (HBV) infection. Injection of a covalently linked construct, composed of a lipidated tetanus toxoid helper peptide and an HLA-A2-restricted HBV core CTL epitope, appeared to be both safe and capable of inducing an HBV-specific CTL response. This was detected by lysis of both peptide-pulsed and HBV-infected HLA-A2$^+$ target cells *in vitro* [38].

The first clinical results of vaccination with defined tumour-associated antigens have recently been observed in patients suffering from melanoma or B cell lymphoma. Although not the initial goal of a phase I/II trial, subcutaneous administration of a peptide representing an HLA-A1-restricted MAGE-3 epitope in PBS, resulted in tumour regressions in three melanoma patients [74]. However, no evidence was obtained for the presence of anti-MAGE-3 T cell activity in these patients. Therefore, the mechanism causing the tumour regression remains as yet unexplained. Alternatively, MAGE-1-directed, tumour-specific CTL were detected in another study consisting of three patients with advanced metastatic melanoma that had been vaccinated with autologous APC pulsed with an HLA-A1-binding MAGE-1 peptide [75]. Despite the presence of anti-tumour CTL, these patients did not show major therapeutic responses, possibly due to the advanced stage of the disease. Finally, clinical responses as well as concomittant anti-tumour T cell-mediated immunity have been observed in three patients with follicular B cell lymphoma after intravenous infusion with autologous dendritic cells pulsed *in vitro* with the patients' tumour-specific idiotype protein [76]. These results indicate that tumour regression may have been mediated by tumour-specific T cells that are activated by vaccination with the specific tumour antigen. In cervical carcinoma patients, several clinical trials have been initiated that aim at inducing or enhancing T cell-mediated immunity against HPV. These trials are based on immunization with i) two HLA-A*0201-restricted HPV 16 E7- encoded peptides administered in combination with a panDR-binding T helper epitope emulsified in an IFA-like adjuvant (University Hospital, Leiden, The Netherlands, ii) recombinant vaccinia virus encoding modified forms of HPV16 and 18 E6 and E7 protein sequences (University of Wales, Cardiff, UK); and iii) an HPV 16 E7 fusion protein (Queensland University, Brisbane, Australia).

After repeated injection with the HPV 16 E7 peptide-based vaccine, two patients have displayed stable disease for over one year so far. This was accompanied by incidentally observed local infiltration of T cells at the site of vaccination, and a proliferative response to the helper peptide included in one patient (M.R., R.B., M.K., C.M., unpublished observations). Furthermore, a single dose of a recombinant vaccinia virus encoding modified forms of the HPV 16 and 18 E6 and E7 protein sequences resulted in a tumour free status of two patients with cervical carcinoma up to 21 months after vaccination. HPV 18 E6/7-specific CTL were detected in one patient. However, it is difficult to envisage that these T cells were responsible for tumour regression since the tumour biopsy sample of this patient did not contain HPV 18 DNA and the E6 and E7 proteins of HPV 16 and 18 display little homology [77]. Nonetheless, these first results of these cervical carcinoma and other tumour immunotherapy trials are both encouraging and instructive for further anti-tumour vaccine development. In several (ongoing) vaccination trials, including our own, clinical effects were observed after vaccination without detectable T cell reactivity against tumour antigens. The source of responding cells, the detection methods used, and the *in vitro* restimulation protocols followed, may have been not suitable for detection of T cell responses in these settings. Most studies so far have used PBMC, while the effective T cells may reside in the tumours or in the lymph nodes. Moreover, both the immune status and tumour burden of the patients at start of vaccination are important for evaluation of the outcome. These factors do not necessarily hamper prospects for anti-cancer immunotherapy, but rather stress the importance of designing reliable methods to assess effectiveness of immunotherapy in patients.

Acknowledgements

In part, these studies were funded by the Dutch Cancer Foundation (grants RUL 93-588, 95-1089) and by the National Institute of Health of the USA (grant 1RO1 CA57933 to M.K.).

Abbreviations

Ad5E1	adenovirus type 5 early region 1
APC	antigen presenting cell(s)
DC	dendritic cell(s)
E	(virus) early region encoded
CTL	cytotoxic T lymphocyte(s)
HBV	hepatitis B virus
HLA	human leukocyte antigen
HPV	human papillomavirus
(IFA) CFA	(in)complete Freunds adjuvant
LCMV	lymphocytic choriomeningitis virus
MHC	major histocompatibility complex
PBMC	peripheral blood mononuclear cells

References

1. F.I.G.O. Carcinoma of the cervix. In: Petterson F (ed). Annual report on the results of treatment in gynaecological cancer. Stockholm, Sweden 1994;22:51-64.
2. Toes REM, Offringa R, Feltkamp MCW, et al.Tumour rejection antigens and tumour specific cytotoxic T lymphocytes. Behring Inst Mitt 1994;94:72-86.
3. Van Pel A,Van der Bruggen P, Coulie PG, et al. Genes coding for tumour antigens recognized by cytolytic T lymphocytes. Immunol Rev 1995;145:229-50.
4. Cheever MA, Disis ML, Bernhard H, et al. Immunity to oncogenic proteins. Immunol Rev, 1995;145:33-59.
5. Toes REM, Feltkamp MCW, Ressing ME, et al. Cellular immunity against DNA tumour viruses: Possibilities for peptide-based vaccines and immune escape. Biochem Soc Trans 1995;23:692-96.
6. Feltkamp MCW, Melief CJM, Kast WM. Peptide-specific cytotoxic T lymphocytes directed against viral oncogene products. In: Dalgleish, Browning (eds). Cambridge Cancer Studies, Tumour Immunology 1996:126-52.
7. Boon T, Van der Bruggen P. Human tumour antigens recognized by T lymphocytes. J Exp Med 1996;183:725-29.
8. Zur Hausen H. Viruses in human cancer. Science 1991;254:1167-72.
9. Masucci MG. Viral immunopathology of human tumors. Curr Opin Immunol, 1993;5: 693-700.
10. Zur Hausen H. Human papillomavirus in the pathogenesis of anogenital cancer. Virology 1991;184:9-13.
11. Seedorf K, Oltersdorf T, Krämmer G, Röwekamp W. Identification of early proteins of the human papillomaviruses type 16 (HPV16) and type 18 (HPV18) in cervical carcinoma cells. EMBO J 1987;6:139-44.
12. Von Knebel Doeberitz M, Bauknecht T, Bartsch D, Zur Hausen H. Influence of chromosomal integration on glucocorticoid-regulated transcription of growth-stimulating papillomavirus genes E6 and E7 in cervical carcinoma cells. Proc Natl Acad Sci USA 1991;88:1411-15.
13. Kast WM, Feltkamp MCW, Ressing ME, Vierboom MPM, Brandt RMP, Melief CJM. Cellular immunity against human papillomavirus associated cervical cancer. Semin Virol 1996;7:117-23.
14. Van den Eynde B, Lethé B, van Pel A, de Plaen E, Boon T. The gene coding for a

major tumour rejection antigen of tumour P815 is identical to the normal gene of syngeneic DBA/2 mice. J Exp Med 1991;173:1373-84.
15. Skipper J, Stauss HJ. Identification of two cytotoxic T lymphocyte- recognized epitopes in the Ras protein. J Exp Med 1993;177:1493-98.
16. Abrams SI, Stanziale SF, Lunin SD, Zaremba S, Schlom J. Identification of overlapping epitopes in mutant Ras oncogene peptides that activate CD4+ and CD8+ T cell responses. Eur J Immunol 1996;26:435-43.
17. Noguchi Y, Richards EC, Chen Y-T, Old LJ. Influence of interleukin 12 on p53 peptide vaccination against established Meth A sarcoma. Proc Natl Acad Sci USA 1995;92: 2219-23.
18. Boon T, Cerottini J-C, Van den Eynde B, Van der Bruggen P, Van Pel A. Tumor antigens recognized by T lymphocytes. Ann Rev Immunol, 1994;12:337-65.
19. Greenberg PD. Adoptive T cell therapy of tumors: mechanisms operative in the recognition and elimination of tumour cells. Adv Immunol 1991;49:281-355.
20. Melief CJM. Tumour eradication by adoptive transfer of cytotoxic T lymphocytes. Adv Cancer Res, 1992;58:143-75.
21. Rosenberg SA, Yannelli JR, Yang J-C, et al. Treatment of patients with metastatic melanoma with autologous tumor-infiltrating lymphocytes and interleukin-2. J Natl Cancer Inst 1994;15:1159-66.
22. Benton C, Shahidullah H, Hunter JAA. Human papillomavirus in the immunosuppressed. Papillomavirus Report 1992;3:23-6.
23. Apple RJ, Erlich HA, Klitz W, Manos MM, Becker TM Wheeler CM. HLA DR-DQ associations with cervical carcinoma show papillomavirus type-specificity. Nat Genet 1994;6:157-62.
24. Bouwes Bavinck JN, Gissman L, Claas FHJ, et al. Relation between skin cancer, humoral responses to human papillomaviruses, and MHC class II molecules in renal transplant patients. J Immunol 1993;151:1579-86.
25. Apple RJ, Becker TM, Wheeler CM, Erlich HA. Comparison of human leukocyte antigen DR-DQ disease associations found with cervical dysplasia and invasive cervical carcinoma. J Natl Cancer Inst 1995:87:427-36.
26. Ellis JRM., Keating PJ, Baird J, et al. The association of an HPV 16 oncogene variant with HLA-B7 has implications for vaccine design in cervical cancer. Nature Med 1995; 1:464-70.
27. Glew SS, Stern PL, Davidson JA, Dyer PA. HLA antigens and cervical carcinoma. Nature 1992;356:22.
28. Connor ME, Stern PL, Loss of MHC class I expression in cervical carcinomas. Int J Cancer 1990;46:1029-34.
29. Cromme FV, Airey J, Heemels MT, et al. Loss of transporter protein, encoded by the TAP-1 gene, is highly correlated with loss of HLA expression in cervical carcinomas. J Exp Med 1994;179:335-40.
30. Honma S, Tsukada S, Honda S, et al. Biological-clinical significance of selective loss of HLA class I allelic product expression in squamous cell carcinoma of the uterine cervix. Int J Cancer 1994;57:650-55.
31. Ferenzy A, Mitoa M, Nagai N, Silverstein SJ, Crum CP. Latent papillomavirus and recurring genital warts. N Engl J Med 1985;313:784-88.
32. Rogozinsky TT, Jablonska S, Jarzabek-Chorzelska M. Role of cell-mediated immunity in spontaneous regression of planar warts. Int J Dermat 1988;27:322-26.
33. Kast WM, Roux L, Curren J, et al. Protection against lethal Sendai virus infection by *in vivo* priming of virus-specific cytotoxic T lymphocytes with an unbound peptide. Proc Natl Acad Sci USA 1991;88:223-87.
34. Schulz M, Zinkernagel RM, Hengartner H. Peptide-induced antiviral protection by

cytotoxic T cells. Proc Natl Acad Sci USA 1991;88:991-93.
35. Schild H, Norda M, Deres K, et al. Fine specificity of cytotoxic T lymphocytes primed *in vivo* either with virus or synthetic lipopeptide vaccine or primed *in vitro* with peptide. J Exp Med 1991;174:1665-68.
36. Reinholdsson-Ljunggren G, Ramqvist T, Åhrlund-Richter L, Dalianis T. Immunization against polyoma tumours with synthetic peptides derived from the sequences of middle- and large-T antigens. Int J Cancer 1992;50:142-46.
37. Minev BR, McFarland BJ, Spiess PJ, Rosenberg SA, Restifo NP. Insertion signal sequence fused to minimal peptides elicits specific CD8+ T-cell responses and prolongs survival of thymoma-bearing mice. Cancer Res 1994;54:4155-6l.
38. Vitiello A, Ishioka G, Grey HM, et al. Development of a lipopeptide-based therapeutic vaccine to treat chronic HBV infection. I. Induction of a primary cytotoxic T lymphocyte response in humans. J Cin Invest 1995;95:341-49.
39. Mayordomo JI, Zitvogel L, Tjandrawan T, Lotze MT, Storkus WJ. Dendritic cells presenting tumour peptide epitopes stimulate effective anti-tumour CTL *in vitro* and *in vivo*. In: Maio (ed). Immunology of human melanoma. Series Biomedical and Health Research 1996;12:153-63.
40. Feltkamp MCW, Smits HL, Vierboom MPM, et al. Vaccination with a cytotoxic T lymphocyte epitope-containing peptide protects against a tumour induced by human papillomavirus type 16-transformed cells. Eur J Immunol 1993;23:2242-49.
41. Feltkamp MCW, Vreugdenhil GR, Vierboom MPM, et al. CTL raised against a subdominant epitope offered as a synthetic peptide eradicate human papillomavirus type 16-induced tumours. Eur J Immunol 1995;25:2638-42.
42. Mayordomo JI, Zorina T, Storkus WJ, et al. Bone marrow-derived dendritic cells pulsed with synthetic tumour peptides elicit protective and therapeutic antitumour immunity. Nature Med 1995;1:1297-1302.
43. Mayordomo JI, Loftus DJ, Sakamoto H, et al. Therapy of murine tumours with p53 wild-type and mutant sequence peptide-based vaccines. J Exp Med 1996;183:1357-65.
44. Mandelboim O, Vadai E, Fridkin M, et al. Regression of established murine carcinoma metastases following vaccination with tumour-associated antigen peptides. Nature Med 1995;1:1179-83.
45. Aichele P, Kyburz D, Ohashi PS, et al. Peptide-induced T-cell tolerance to prevent autoimmune diabetes in a transgenic mouse model. Proc Natl Acad Sci USA 1994; 91:444-48.
46. Aichele P, Brduscha-Riem K, Zinkernagel RM, Hengartner H, Pircher H. T cell priming versus T cell tolerance induced by synthetic peptides. J Exp Med 1995;182: 261-66.
47. Kast WM, Offringa R, Peters PJ, et al. Eradication of Adenovirus E1-induced tumours by EIA-specific cytotoxic T lymphocytes. Cell 1989;59:603-14.
48. Toes REM, Offringa R, Blom HJJ, et al. An adenovirus type 5 early region 1B-encoded CTL epitope-mediating tumour eradication by CTL clones is down-modulated by an activated ras oncogene. J Immunol 1995;154:3396-405.
49. Toes REM, Offringa R, Blom RJJ, Melief CJM, Kast WM. Peptide vaccination can lead to enhanced tumour growth through specific T-cell tolerance induction. Proc Natl Acad Sci USA 1996;93:7855-60.
50. Toes REM, Blom RJJ, Offringa R, Kast WM, Melief CJM. Enhanced tumour outgrowth after peptide vaccination. Functional deletion of tumour-specific CTL induced by peptide vaccination can lead to the inability to reject tumours. J Immunol 1996;156: 3911-18.
5l. Bevan MJ. Antigen presentation to cytotoxic T lymphocytes *in vivo*. J Exp Med 1995; 182:639-4l.
52. Flamand V, Sornasse T, Thielemans K. Murine dendritic cells pulsed *in vitro* with

tumour antigen induce tumour resistance *in vivo*. Eur J Immunol 1994;24:605-10.
53. Paglia P, Chiodoni C, Rodolfo M, Colombo MP. Murine dendritic cells loaded *in vitro* with soluble protein prime cytotoxic T lymphocytes against tumour antigen *in vivo*. J Exp Med 1996;183:317-22.
54. Zitvogel L, Mayordomo JI, Tjandrawan T, et al. Therapy of murine tumours with tumour peptide-pulsed dendritic cells: dependence of T cells, B7 costimulation, and T helper cell l-associated cytokines. J Exp Med 1996;183:87-97.
55. Pardoll DM. New strategies for enhancing the immunogenicity of tumours. Curr Opin Immunol 1993;5:719-25.
56. Pardoll DM. Paracrine cytokine adjuvants in cancer immunotherapy. Ann Rev Immunol 1995;13:399-415.
57. Seung S, Urban JL, Schreiber HA. Tumour escape variant that has lost one major histocompatibility complex class I restriction element induces specific CD8+ T cells to an antigen that no longer serves as a target. J Exp Med 1993;178:933-40.
58. Huang AYC, Golumbek P, Ahmadzadeh M, Jaffee E, Pardoll D, Levitsky H. Role of bone marrow-derived cells in presenting MHC class I-restricted tumour antigens. Science 1994;264:961-65.
59. Toes REM, Blom RJJ, Van der Voort EIH, Offringa R, Melief CJM, Kast WM. Protective anti-tumour immunity induced by immunization with completely allogeneic tumour cells. Cancer Res 1996;56:3782-87.
60. Le A-XT, Bernhard EJ, Holterman MJ, et al. Cytotoxic T cell responses in HLA-A2.1 transgenic mice: recognition of HLA alloantigens and utilization of HLA-A2.1 as a restriction element. J Immunol 1989;142:1366-71.
61. Vitiello A, Marchesini D, Furze JSSL, Chesnut RW. Analysis of the HLA-restricted influenza-specific cytotoxic T lymphocyte response in transgenic mice carrying a chimeric human-mouse class I major histocompatibility complex. J Exp Med 1991;173:1007-15.
62. Engelhard VH, Lacy E, Ridge JP. Influenza A-specific, HLA-A2.1- restricted cytotoxic T lymphocytes from HLA-A2.1 transgenic mice recognize fragments of the M1 protein. J Immunol 1991;146:1226-32.
63. Newberg MH, Ridge JP, Vining DR, Salter RD, Engelhard VH. Species specificity in the interaction of CD8 with the alpha 3 domain of MHC class I molecules. J Immunol 1992;149:136-42.
64. Man S, Ridge JP, Engelhard VH. Diversity and dominance among TCR recognizing HLA-A2.1+ influenza matrix peptide in human MHC class I transgenic mice. J Immunol 1994;153:4458-67.
65. Lehner PJ, Wang ECY, Moss PAH, et al. Human HLA-A*0201-restricted cytotoxic T lymphocyte recognition of influenza A is dominated by T cells bearing the V beta 17 gene segment. J Exp Med 1995;181:79-91.
66. Shirai M, Arichi T, Nishioka M, et al. CTL responses of HLA-A2.1-transgenic mice specific for hepatitis C viral peptides predict epitopes for CTL of humans carrying HLA-2.1. J Immunol 1995;154:2733-42.
67. Sette A, Vitiello A, Reherman B, et al. The relationship between class I binding affinity and immunogenicity of potential cytotoxic T cell epitopes. J Immunol 1994;153:5586-92.
68. Ressing ME, Sette A, Brandt RMP, et al. Human CTL epitopes encoded human papillomavirus type 16 E6 and E7 identified through *in vivo* and *in vitro* immunogenicity studies of HLA-A*0201-binding peptides. J Immunol 1995;154:5934-43.
69. Theobald M, Biggs J, Dittmer D, Levine AJ, Sherman LA. Targeting p53 as a general tumour antigen. Proc Natl Acad Sci USA 1995;92:11993-97.
70. Wentworth PA, Vitiello A, Sidney J, et al. Differences and similarities in the A2.1-

restricted cytotoxic T cell repertoire in humans and human leukocyte antigen-transgenic mice. Eur J Immunol 1996;26:97-101.

71. Kast WM, Brandt RMP, Drijfhout JW, Melief CJM. Human leukocyte antigen-A2.1 restricted candidate cytotoxic T lymphocyte epitopes of human papillomavirus type 16 E6 and E7 proteins identified by using the processing-defective human cell line T2. J Immunother 1993;14:115-20.
72. Kast WM, Brandt RMP, Sidney J, et al. Role of HLA-A motifs in identification of potential CTL epitopes in human papillomavirus type 16 E6 and E7 proteins. J Immunol 1994;152:3904-12.
73. Ressing ME, van Driel WJ, Celis E, et al. Occasional memory cytotoxic T-cell responses of patients with human papillomavirus type 16-positive cervical lesions against a human leukocyte antigen-A*0201-restricted E7-encoded epitope. Cancer Res 1996; 56:582-88.
74. Merchand M, Weynants P, Rankin E, et al. Tumour regression responses in melanoma patients treated with a peptide encoded by gene MAGE-3. Int J Cancer 1995;63:883-85.
75. Mukherji B, Chakraborty NG, Yamasaki S, et al. Induction of antigen-specific cytolytic T cells *in situ* in human melanoma by immunization with synthetic peptide-pulsed autologous antigen presenting cells. Proc Natl Acad Sci USA 1995;92:8078-82.
76. Hsu FJ, Benike C, Fagnoni F, et al. Vaccination of patients with B-cell lymphoma using autologous antigen-pulsed dendritic cells. Nature Med 1996;2:52-82.
77. Borysiewicz LK, Fiander A, Nimako M, et al. A recombinant vaccinia virus encoding human papillomavirus types 16 and 18, E6 and E7 proteins as immunotherapy for cervical cancer. Lancet 1996;347:1523-27.

CYTOKINES IN THE TREATMENT OF INFECTION

D.C. Dale

Introduction

It is now well accepted that host defense mechanisms, both cellular and humoral, are regulated by a family of cytokines, interleukins and colony-stimulating factors (CSFs). Control of antibody production and humoral immunity including antigen processing, T-cell and B-cell responses and the proliferation of plasma cells are under the control of Interleukin-2 (IL-2) through IL-17. Naturally occurring diseases and gene "knockout" experiments in mice clearly indicate the essential roles for some of these factors and their receptors in maintaining humoral immunity [1]. Similarly, cellular immunity, largely mediated through T-cells, is under the control of the interleukins, and mediated through specific cell surface receptors for these factors. Although our understanding of interleukins in humoral and cellular host defense mechanisms is advancing rapidly, clinical applications of interleukins to modify *in vivo* lymphocyte mediated responses is still largely at the investigative stage. Interesting potential clinical applications include the use of IL-2 to treat HIV infected individuals [2], the use of autologous IL-2 expanded cells for prevention of cytomegalovirus infections in bone marrow transplant patients [3], and potential applications of IL-10 to modify the suppressor/helper functions of lymphocytes in a variety of inflammatory and infectious diseases [4]. The interferons, well characterized cytokines produced in response to many viral infections, can also be used pharmacologically to modify the course of hepatitis B, hepatitis C, and some other infections as outlined in recent reviews [5,6].

The supply, deployment and function of the phagocytic cells of the host defense system is also under the control of cytokines [7]. The occurrence and outcome for most bacterial, fungal and parasitic infections depends upon the availability and function of these cells, i.e., neutrophils, eosinophils, monocytes and the fixed mononuclear phagocytes found in the spleen, liver, lungs and other tissues. These cells are critical for prevention of infection from micro-organisms found normally on body surfaces, as well as for protection from more invasive and pathogenic organisms. The cytokines regulating phagocyte development and function now have several practical applications for the prevention and treatment of infections.

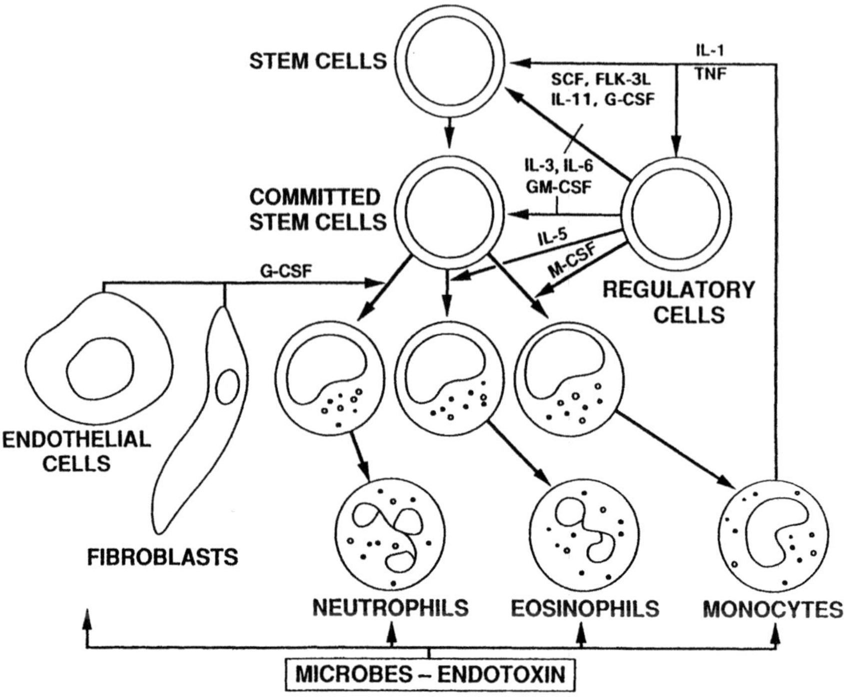

Figure 1. Model for the regulation of neutrophil, eosinophil and monocyte production in infectious diseases. At sites of infection, monocytes and tissue macrophages produce long range factors such as interleukin-1 (IL-1) and tumour necrosis factor (TNF). These factors activate haematopoietic stem cells and other regulatory cells of the marrow (T lymphocytes and stromal cells) to produce the factors stimulating the early phases of haematopoiesis. Microbes and endotoxin also increase the production of G-CSF, M-CSF and IL-6, which increase production and blood levels of neutrophils, monocytes and esosinophils respectively.

Cytokine regulation of phagocyte production and function

All types of phagocytes derive from the common haematopoietic stem cells and production of phagocytes is governed by haematopoietic growth factors, some of which are called colony-stimulating factors. From the discovery of these factors in the 1960s to the present, much interest has focused on *in vivo* and *in vitro* studies of how these factors are affected by inflammation, infection and exposure of cells or whole organisms to bacterial lipopolysaccharide (LPS) or endotoxin [8,9]. For instance, the discovery of the key regulatory cytokine for neutrophil production, granulocyte colony-stimulating factor (G-CSF), came from experiments in mice showing that this factor, in contrast to granulocyte macrophage colony-stimulating factor (GM-CSF), was found in high concentrations in serum or plasma from mice soon after injection of LPS [10,11].

Our current general understanding of the role of cytokines and colony-stimulating factors in influencing phagocyte production is illustrated in Figure 1. There are several key features of this schema:

1. Production of mature cells is governed by "early-acting" factors and "late-acting"" factors. The factors affecting the early phases of haematopoiesis, e.g., IL-3, IL-11, SCF and FLK-3 ligand, influence production of erythrocytes and platelets, as well as leukocytes. Receptors for these cytokines are not present on mature cells. In this schema, tumour necrosis factor (TNF) and IL-1 may serve as long range regulators interacting with these factors in stimulating early haematopoietic cell proliferation in inflammatory conditions [12].

2. Some cytokines have both early and late effects, such as G-CSF and GM-CSF. Both immature and mature cells of the neutrophilic series have receptors for both of these cytokines. Monocytes and eosinophils have GM-CSF receptors [13].

3. The late-acting factors, G-CSF, M-CSF and IL-5 specifically govern the late phases of neutrophil, monocyte and eosinophil production respectively. Levels of G-CSF and M-CSF, as well as IL-6, are increased with inflammation and decreased as inflammation resolves [14,15].

4. Maintenance of the integrity of the phagocytic system undoubtedly involves the cooperation of all of these cytokines but redundancies may exist both for protective and for evolutionary reasons [16].

Cytokine responses in infections

Acute bacterial infections or injection of LPS induces the expression of several well characterized cytokines, including tumour necrosis factor, IL-1 and IL-6 [17-19]. The time course for these acute phase reactants is well described. Parallel studies of colony-stimulating factor responses with acute infection and after LPS administration have shown that G-CSF and M-CSF, but not GM-CSF, increase with infections or after LPS administration, both in animals and in man [15,20]. In comparison to baseline levels, the degree of increase in G-CSF levels for patients in septic shock and after high dose LPS administration is quite large [21,22]. In clinical studies the increases in G-CSF correlate with the severity of infection, the presence of bacteremia, specifically Gram-negative bacteremia, and reductions in renal function [15]. After acute infection, G-CSF fall back to normal within a few days [23].

Because serum or plasma levels of the cytokines governing haematopoiesis are very low or undetectable with current assay systems, it has been difficult to identify conditions which cause deficiencies of the factors. Gene deletion or "knockout" experiments, however, clearly show that deficiencies of G-CSF result in neutropenia with increased susceptibility to infection [24]. A similar G-CSF-deficiency state has been produced in dogs through repeated administration of recombinant human G-CSF, with resulting production of cross-reacting antibodies to canine G-

CSF [25]. A neutropenic state can also be induced by infusion of anti-G-CSF antibodies [25]. It is not yet known, however, if any clinical conditions associated with neutropenia are due to a deficiency of G-CSF or any other haematopoietic growth factor. Interestingly, animals made deficient in GM-CSF through embryonal stem cell disruption are not neutropenic; they have proteinaceous accumulations in the lung, resembling the disease alveolar proteinosis [26].

Studies of the effects of CSF administration in normal human subiects

The physiological effects of CSF administration to normal subjects has provided an important basis for trials utilizing these factors for the treatment of infections in man. Normal volunteers given G-CSF (30 µg or 300 µg/day) daily for 14 days had increases in neutrophil production approximately seven-fold [27]. Marrow studies showed an increase in early precursor cell proliferation and hastening of the transit of cells through the marrow post-mitotic pool into the blood [27]. In addition, G-CSF affects primary granule formation, increases the leukocyte alkaline phosphatase scores, primes cells for an enhanced metabolic burst as reflected by chemiluminescence assays, enhances superoxide production and enhances the killing of bacteria and fungi [28]. Surface expression of CD-14 and CD-64 are also increased, indicating that the cells produced in response to G-CSF may have enhanced interactions with foreign cells and bacterial products [28-31]. When G-CSF is administered to healthy volunteers *in vivo* it initially induces increased expression of CD-llbl8, but longer administration (5 days) causes down-regulation of this expression. There is also increased and then decreased expression of LAM-1 (leukocyte adhesion molecule-1, or L-selectin) [28]. G-CSF prolongs the life of neutrophils both *in vitro* and *in vivo* through suppression of the process of apoptosis, or programmed cell death [27,32]. Thus, G-CSF causes neutrophilia, both in pharmacologically and naturally-occurring inflammatory states. In addition, this cytokine mobilizes neutrophils prepared to focus their armamentarium of anti-bacterial substances at sites of infection.

Similar studies of GM-CSF show that it also stimulates neutrophil production and increases marrow and blood eosinophils and monocytes [33,34, Dale et al, unpublished observations]. In a dose of 250 µg/m2 given for 14 days in a similar protocol to that used for the above studies with G-CSF, it was observed to be somewhat less potent in inducing neutrophilia than G-CSF.

Other effects are similar, however, in priming neutrophils for enhanced metabolic response to exposure to bacteria and foreign particles. In normal subjects, as well as most clinical trials, GM-CSF has many more associated adverse effects than G-CSF.

Preclinical applications of cytokines for the treatment of infections

Clinical Applications

Beginning in the late 1980s several investigators began using haematopoietic cytokines for the treatment of animals with experimental infections. These preclinical studies have involved mice, rats, guinea pigs, rabbits, dogs and primates, and include animals with normal haematopoiesis as well as those with drug or radiation-induced myelosuppression [28]. Models studied include sepsis, both in neonates [35-37] and adults [38-40], pneumonia [41,42], burns [43,44], and intramuscular infections [45]. The largest number of studies have involved the use of G-CSF because of its availability and its potent effects on neutrophil formation. Several general principals have been learned from these experiments. These are:

1. The neutrophilia which develops in most experimental infections is not the maximal response. G-CSF administration to haematologically intact animals with infections will generally further elevate blood neutrophils.

2. The timing of treatment is important. The most favorable results are observed when treatment precedes infection or follows soon after infection. With G-CSF, GM-CSF or other haematopoietic cytokines, the blood neutrophil count rises for several days after beginning the drug to reach a new plateau level. The effect of these cytokines on the quality, as well as the quantity of cells produced undoubtedly also affects outcome.

3. Most experiments involve the use of cytokines with antibiotics, but favorable effects also have been observed in animals treated with G-CSF without concomitant antibiotic administration. It is not yet clear if antibiotics which are concentrated intracellularly, such as rifampin, chloramphenicol, azithromycin, etc., are more effective than drugs such as the penicillins and cephalosporins, which are not actively taken up by phagocytes.

4. Increasing the body' s production of neutrophils and the supply of cells available to migrate to a site of infection increases the tissue inflammatory response. In addition, some studies have shown that the clearance of organisms from tissues is enhanced through the use of G-CSF to increase the neutrophil supply.

5. In studies with G-CSF the induction of neutrophilia and an increase in the neutrophil response is not associated with tissue injury. For example, in animals with pneumonia, G-CSF treatment did not directly cause lung injury or the acute respiratory distress syndrome (ARDS) [46-48]. Thus, preclinical trials suggested that the use of G-CSF for treatment of infections would be both safe and efficacious.

Clinical trials

Most of our information on the use of cytokines for the treatment of infections comes from studies of G-CSF and GM-CSF. In patients with neutropenia due to cancer chemotherapy or bone marrow transplantation, these cytokines can accelerate neutrophil recovery, minimizing the duration of severe neutropenia, and reduce the occurrence and severity of infections [49]. In this regard, the results of studies are not uniform, in part related to the relative low frequency of documented infections in some of these studies. In patients with congenital, cyclic or idiopathic neutropenia, clinical trials have shown that G-CSF increases blood neutrophils and reduces the occurrence of fever, oropharyngeal inflammation, and infections [50]. To attain these benefits, daily or alternate day therapy is required. Long term treatment of these patients with G-CSF has provided continuing benefit without loss of efficacy in almost all patients. Antibody formation to G-CSF or changes in marrow responsiveness has generally not occurred. In a few patients with congenital neutropenia, however, an underlying propensity for conversion to myelodysplasia and acute myeloid leukemia has been recognized and the frequency and significance of these findings is under continued investigation. GM-CSF has been investigated as a long term treatment in a few patients, but is generally not used because of its side effects. No other haematopoietic cytokines have thus far been proven to be useful for the treatment of acute or chronic neutropenia.

Another important application of the haematopoietic cytokines is for the treatment of neutropenia associated with HIV infection [51]. The first major clinical trial of GM-CSF was in men with HIV infection. This initial trial and numerous subsequent trials have demonstrated that HIV positive patients with neutropenia due to viral infection or as a complication of anti-viral chemotherapy or cancer chemotherapy will respond to GM-CSF or G-CSF to increase their blood neutrophil counts. This responsiveness is retained even in the late stages of HIV infection. Accumulating data suggests that G-CSF and GM-CSF affects neutrophils in HIV infected individuals by several mechanisms: enhanced production, reduced cell loss through apoptosis and improvement in neutrophil function. The use of G-CSF or GM-CSF for neutropenia in HIV positive patients remains controversial, however, because of the lack of well designed control trials establishing clinical benefit. Some recent evidence suggests that G-CSF may reduce the occurrence of bacterial infections in the most neutropenic of these patients [52]. G-CSF is used more widely than GM-CSF to maintain neutrophil levels so that HIV positive individuals can receive anti-viral chemotherapy.

CSF treatment of infections of non-neutropenic infections

Based upon experience with G-CSF administration for the prevention and treatment of infections in neutropenic patients and the preclinical studies in animals, the first major treatment trials of G-CSF for infections in non-neutropenic patients were begun in individuals with community-acquired pneumonia. The initial studies established that even with elevation of the blood neutrophil counts to 50 to 100×10^9/L there was no apparent adverse effect on lung function or blood oxygenation [53]. Subsequently a large randomized trial was conducted in the U.S. and Australia, testing whether G-CSF is a useful adjunct to conventional antibiotic therapy or severely ill patients with community-acquired pneumonia [54]. Patients enrolled in this trial tended to be elderly patients with other health problems predisposing them to a more prolonged hospital course, need for intravenous antibiotics and greater likelihood of secondary complications. The patients were not sufficiently ill to be classified as having septic shock. In this trial the primary endpoint was the time to resolution of fever, tachypnea, hypoxia and pneumonia by x-ray examination. Although the time to this endpoint was not decreased for the study population as a whole, the more severely ill patients in the trial, particularly those with multi-lobar pneumonia, appeared to benefit from G-CSF treatment. In addition, the study also showed that G-CSF treatment reduced the rate of multi-organ failure, acute respiratory distress syndrome, and development of septic shock. Resolution of pulmonary infiltrates by x-ray was also more rapid in the G-CSF treated group. Comparing the G-CSF treated patients to the placebo groups, several other interesting and important observations were made. The median of three-fold increase in blood neutrophils was not associated with the worsening of pulmonary status. Neutrophil infiltration of other tissues as could be determined by clinical evaluation was not observed and there were very few side effects of this therapy. Based upon these findings, particularly the apparent benefit for the sicker individuals, further studies of G-CSF treatment in pneumonia are under way. To date there have been limited trials of GM-CSF for the treatment of infections in man. There is some promising data for adjunctive use of GM-CSF in the treatment of leishmaniasis [55-57]. Thus far, no clear conclusions have come from these trials.

Conclusion

Normal host defense mechanisms are governed by the production of cytokines, interleukins, and the colony-stimulating factors. Recent research has delineated many important mechanisms and potential applications for cytokines for enhancing host defenses to prevent or treat infection. One of the most promising applications is in the use of the cytokines which influence haematopoiesis and the regulation and deployment of phagocytes. Among these cytokines, G-CSF is the most promising candidate, because of its unique role in regulating and maintaining the blood neutrophil count. Physiological studies, preclinical trials and clinical studies in both neutropenic and non-neutropenic patients suggest that G-CSF is useful for prevention of infections in several circumstances and may prove useful as an adjunct for antibiotics, particularly for patients with severe infections. Clinical trials are now underway testing this hypothesis.

References

1. Murray R. Physiologic roles of interleukin-2, interleukin-4, and interleukin-7. Cur Opn Hematol 1996;3:230-34.
2. Kovacs JA, Baseler M, Dewar RJ et al. Increases in CD4 T lymphocytes with intermittent courses of interleukin-2 in patients with human immunodeficiency virus infection. N Engl J Med 1995;332:567-75.
3. Walter EA, Greenberg PD, Gilbert MJ et al. Reconstitution of cellular immunity against cytomegalovirus in recipients of allogeneic bone marrow by transfer of T-cell clones from the donor. N Engl J Med 1995;333:1038-44.
4. Geissler K. Current status of clinical development of interleukin-10. Cur Opn Hematol 1996;3:203-08.
5. Gallin JI, Farber JM, Holland SM, Nutman TB. Interferon-gamma in the management of infectious diseases. Ann Intern Med 1995;123:216-24.
6. Hoofnagle JH. Therapy of acute and chronic viral hepatitis. Adv Intern Med 1994; 39:241-75.
7. Sachs L. The control of hematopoiesis and leukemia: From basic biology to the clinic. Proc Natl Acad Sci USA 1996;93:4742-49.

8. Metcalf D. The role of the colony-stimulating factors in resistance to acute infections. Immunol Cell Biol 1987;65(Pt. 1):35-43.
9. Cheers C, Haigh AM, Kelso A, et al. Production of colony-stimulating factors (CSFs) during infection: Separate determinations of macrophage-, granulocyte-, and multi-CSFs. Infection and Immunity 1988;56:247-51.
10. Nicola NA, Metcalf D, Johnson GR, Burgess AW. Separation of functionally distinct human granulocyte-macrophage colony-stimulating factors. Blood 1979;54:614-27.
11. Nicola NA, Metcalf D, Matsumoto M, Johnson GR: Purification of a factor inducing differentiation in murine myelomonocytic leukemia cells. J Biol Chem 1983;258:9017-23.
12. Dinarello CA. Biologic basis for interleukin-1 in disease. Blood 1996;87:2095-147.
13. Lieschke GJ, Burgess AW. Granulocyte colony-stimulating factor and granulocyte-macrophage colony-stimulating factor, parts I and II. N Engl J Med 1992;327:(I)28-35,(II)99-106.
14. Cebon J, Layton J. Measurement and clinical significance of circulating hematopoietic growth factor levels. Curr Opn Hematol 1994;1:228-34.
15. Cebon J, Layton J, Maher D, Morstyn G. Endogenous haemopoietic growth factors in neutropenia and infection. Brit J Haematol 1994;86:265-74.
16. Metcalf D. Hematopoietic regulators: Redundancy or subtlety? Blood 1993;82:3515-23.
17. Hermann JL, Blanchard H, Brunengo P, Lagrange PH. TNF alpha, IL-1 beta and IL-6 plasma levels in neutropenic patients after onset of fever and correlation with the C-reactive protein (CRP) kinetic values. Infection 1994;22:309-15.
18. Gardlund B, Sjolin J, Nilsson A, Roll M, Wickerts CJ, Wretlind B. Plasma levels of cytokines in primary septic shock in humans: Correlation with disease severity. J Infect Dis 1995;172:296-301.
19. Waring PM, Presneill J, Maher DW, et al. Differential alterations in plasma colony-stimulating factor concentrations in meningococcaemia. Clin Exp Immunol 1995;102:501-06.
20. Kuhns DB, Alvord WG, Gallin JI. Increased circulating cytokines, cytokine antagonists, and E-selectin after intravenous administration of endotoxin in humans. J Infec Dis 1995;171:145-52.
21. Taveira Da Silva AMT, Kaulbach HC, Chuidian FS, et al. Brief report: Shock and multiple-organ dysfunction after self-administration of salmonella endotoxin. N Engl J Med 1993;328:1457-60.
22. Dale DC, Lau S, Nash R, Boone T, Osborne W. The effect of endotoxin on serum granulocyte and granulocyte-macrophage colony stimulating factor (G-CSF and GM-CSF) levels in dogs. J Inf Dis 1991;87:704-10.
23. Kawakami M, Tsutsumi H, Kumakawa T, et al. Levels of serum granulocyte colony-stimulating factor in patients with infections. Blood 1990;76:1962-64.
24. Lieschke GJ, Grail D, Hodgson G, et al. Mice lacking granulocyte colony-stimulating factor have chronic neutropenia, granulocyte and macrophage progenitor cell deficiency, and impaired neutrophil mobilization. Blood 1994;84:1737-46.
25. Hammond WP, Csiba E, Canin A, Souza LM, Dale DC. Chronic neutropenia: A new canine model induced by human G-CSF. J Clin Invest 1991;87:704-10.
26. Dranoff G, Crawford AD, Sadelain M, et al. Involvement of granulocyte-macrophage colony-stimulating factor in pulmonary homeostasis. Science 1994;294:713-16.
27. Price TH, Chatta GS, Dale DC. The effect of recombinant granulocyte colony-stimulating factor on neutrophil kinetics in normal young and elderly humans. Blood 1996;88:335-40.
28. Dale DC, Liles WC, Summer W, Nelson S. Granulocyte-colony-stimulating factor:

Role and relationships in infectious diseases. J Inf Dis 1995;172:1061-75.
29. Kerst JM, de Haas M, van der Schoot CE, et al. Recombinant granulocyte colony-stimulating factor administration to healthy volunteers: Induction of immunophenotypically and functionally altered neutrophils via an effect on myeloid progenitor cells. Blood 1993;82:3265-72.
30. Repp R, Valerius T, Sendler A, et al. Neutrophils express the high affinity receptor for IgG (FcγRI; CD64) after *in vivo* application of rhG-CSF. Blood 1991;78:885-89.
31. Kerst JM, van de Winkel JGJ, Evans AH, et al. Granulocyte colony-stimulating factor induces hFcγRI (CD64 antigen)-positive neutrophils via an effect on myeloid precursor cells. Blood 1993;81:1457-64.
32. Colotta F, Re F, Polentarutti N, et al. Modulation of granulocyte survival and programmed cell death by cytokines and bacterial products. Blood 1992;80:2012-20.
33. Aglietta M, Piacibello W, Sanavio F, et al. Kinetics of human hemopoietic cells after *in vivo* administration of granulocyte-macrophage colony-stimulating factor. J Clin Invest 1989;83:551-57.
34. Hill ADK, Naama HA, Calvano SE, Daly JM. The effect of granulocyte-macrophage colony-stimulating factor on myeloid cells and its clinical applications. J Leuko Biol 1995;58:634-42.
35. Cairo MS, Mauss D, Kommareedy S, et al. Prophylactic or simultaneous administration of recombinant human granulocyte colony-stimulating factor in the treatment of group B streptococcal sepsis in neonatal rats. Pediatr Res 1990;27:612-16.
36. Liechty KW, Schibler KR, Ohls RK, et al. The failure of newborn mice infected with Escherichia coli to accelerate neutrophil production correlates with their failure to increase transcripts for granulocyte colony-stimulating factor and interleukin-6. Biol Neonate 1993;64:331-40.
37. Cairo MS, Plunkett JM, Mauss D, van de Ven C. Seven-day administration of recombinant human granulocyte colony-stimulating factor to newborn rats: Modulation of neonatal neutrophilia, myelopoiesis, and group B Streptococcus sepsis. Blood 1990; 76:1788-94.
38. Herbert JC, O'Reilly M, Gamelli RL. Protective effect of recombinant human granulocyte colony-stimulating factor against pneumococcal infections in splenectomized mice. Arch Surg 1990;125:1075-78.
39. Toda H, Murata A, Oka Y, et al. Effect of granulocyte-macrophage colony-stimulating factor on sepsis-induced organ injury in rats. Blood 1994;83:2893-98.
40. Eichacker PQ, Waisman y, Natanson C, et al. Cardiopulmonary effects of granulocyte colony-stimulating factor in a canine model of bacterial sepsis. J Appli Physiol 1994; 77:2366-73.
41. Nelson S, Summer W, Bagby G, et al. Granulocyte colony-stimulating factor enhances pulmonary host defenses in normal and ethanol-treated rats. J Infect Dis 1991;164:901-06.
42. Lister PD, Gentry MJ, Preheim LC. Granulocyte colony-stimulating factor protects control rats but not ethanol-fed rats from fatal pneumococcal pneumonia. J Infect Dis 1993;168:922-26.
43. Mooney DP, Gamelli RL, O'Reilly M, Hebert JC. Recombinant human granulocyte colony-stimulating factor and Pseudomonas burn wound sepsis. Arch Surg 1988;123: 1353-57.
44. Silver GM, Gamelli RL, O' Reilly M. The beneficial effect of granulocyte colony-stimulating factor (G-CSF) on survival after Pseudomonas burn wound infection. Surgery 1989;106:452-56.
45. Jyung RW, Wu L, Pierce GF, Mustoe TA. Granulocyte-macrophage colony-stimulating factor and granulocyte colony-stimulating factor: Differential action on incisional

wound healing. Surgery 1994;115:325-34.

46. Fink MP, O'Sullivan BP, Menconi MJ, et al. Effect of granulocyte colony-stimulating factor on systemic and pulmonary responses to endotoxin in pigs. J Trauma 1993; 34:571-78.
47. Koizumi T, Kubo K, ShinozakiS, et al. Granulocyte colony-stimulating factor does not exacerbate endotoxin-induced lung injury in sheep. Am Rev Respir Dis 1993;148:132-37.
48. Kanazawa M, Ishizaka A, Hasegawa N, et al. Granulocyte colony-stimulating factor does not enhance endotoxin-induced acute lung injury in guinea pigs. Am Rev Respir Dis 1992;145:1030-35.
49. Ozer H (for Am Soc Clin Oncol ad hoc CSSF Guidelines Expert Panel) American Society of Clinical Oncology recommendations for the use of hematopoietic colony-stimulating factors: Evidence-based clinical practice guidelines. J Clin Oncol 1994;12: 2471-508.
50. Dale DC, Bonilla MA, Davis MW, et al. A randomized controlled phase III trial of recombinant human G-CSF for treatment of severe chronic neutropenia. Blood 1993; 81:2496-502.
51. Frumkin L, Dale DC. The role of colony-stimulating factors in HIV disease. The Aids Reader 1996;Nov/Dec185-93.
52. Keiser P, Rademacher S. G-CSF use is associated with decreased bacteremia and increased survival in neutropenic, HIV infected patients. 3rd Conference on retrovirus and opportunistic infections. Washington DC 1996:abstract 518.
53. DeBoisblanc B, Summer WR, Mason C, Shellito J, Andresen J, Nelson S. A phase I trial of granulocyte colony-stimulating factor in severe community-acquired pnemonia Am Rev Resp Dis 1993;147(4):A204.
54. Nelson S, Farkas S, Fotheringham N, Ho H, Mattie T, Movahhed H. Filgrastim in the treatment of hospitalized patients with community acquired pneumonia. Am J Crit Care Med 1996;153:A535.
55. Murray HW, Cervia JS, Hariprashad J, Taylor AP, Stoeckle MY, Hockman H. Effect of granulocyte-macrophage colony-stimulating factor in experimental leishmaniasis. J Clin Invest 1995;95:1183-92.
56. Badar'o R, Nascimento C, Carvalho JS, et al. Granulocyte-macrophage colony-stimulating factor in combination with pentavalent antimony for the treatment of visceral Leishmaniasis. Eur J Clin Microbiol Infect Dis 1994;3:S23-28.
57. Badar'o R, Nascimento C, Carvalho JS, et al. Recombinant human granulocyte-macrophage colony-stimulating factor reverses neutropenia and reduces secondary infections in visceral leishmaniasis. J Infect Dis 1994;170:413-18.

THROMBOPOIETIN: BIOLOGICAL EFFECTS BEYOND MEGAKARYOPOIESIS

K. Kaushansky

Why look for a role of thrombopoietin on non-megakaryocytic lineages?

Since the cloning of thrombopoietin (TPO) in 1994 multiple studies have appeared that establish its critical role in megakaryocyte and platelet production [reviewed in 1]. However, several observations suggest that the haematopoietic effects of the hormone might be greater than initially anticipated. For example, TPO was initially cloned by many groups as the Mpl ligand [2-4], the hormone which bound to the proto-oncogene receptor c-Mpl. This gene, in turn, was cloned as the cellular homologue of *v-mpl* [5], the transforming gene of the murine myeloproliferative leukemia virus (MPLV). As all lineages of haematopoietic development are affected by this disease [6], it was clear from early studies that an autonomously active mpl receptor could signal in multiple cell types, possibly including the haematopoietic stem cell. Along these same lines, expression of *c-mpl* mRNA was detected in a number of fresh leukemic marrow samples, including myeloid, erythroid and undifferentiated subclasses of the disease [7]. A second line of evidence also supports the concept that the primary regulator of megakaryopoiesis might also affect another lineage, namely erythropoiesis. The two lineages display several common properties, including their shared expression of multiple transcription factors (e.g. GATA, NF-E2, SCL) and cell surface receptors (e.g. c-kit, IL-3-R, EPO-R, c-mpl) [8,9]. In addition, we and others have provided clear evidence for a common erythroid/megakaryocytic progenitor cell [CFU-EMk; refs.10,11]. And perhaps most compelling, the introduction of a thymidine kinase gene linked to the "megakaryocyte-specific" glycoprotein IIb promoter into transgenic mice leads to the elimination not only of platelet but also erythrocyte production when this "suicide gene" was activated by feeding gancyclovir [12]. Together, these findings clearly indicate the commonality of erythropoiesis and megakaryopoiesis, and as EPO has been shown to affect megakaryocyte production both *in vitro* and *in vivo* [13,14], suggest that TPO might also augment erythropoiesis. Finally, the role of a "lineage-specific" hormone in the function of primitive haematopoietic cells has already been provided; G-CSF acts in synergy with IL-3 to accelerate the entry of blast cell colony forming cells into the cell cycle [15]. Taken all together these findings argue that TPO might play more of a role in haematopoiesis than initially predicted.

TPO acts in synergy with EPO to promote erythropoiesis

In order to determine whether TPO exerts effects on red cell development we tested whether the hormone, alone or together, affects the growth of erythroid progenitor cells. Alone, TPO failed to induce the growth of either BFU-E or CFU-E. In contrast, in the presence of EPO, the number of both early and late marrow erythroid progenitors was increased two to three fold [16]. However, as these experiments we conducted with whole marrow cells, the effects of TPO may have been indirect. To assess whether TPO directly affects erythropoiesis, Ogawa's lab plucked individual immature erythroid bursts and replated them in the presence of either EPO, TPO or both hormones. The number of both cord blood and marrow derived "secondary BFU-E" increased approximately three-fold in these cultures, providing strong evidence that TPO exerts a direct synergistic effect on erythropoiesis [17].

We next sought to determine whether these *in vitro* erythropoietic properties of TPO correlated with effects *in vivo*. When TPO was administered to normal mice we found that the number of BFU-E increased in the marrow and spleen, but the CFU-E, reticulocyte and mature red cell counts in the animals remained constant (16). These results were not unexpected; whatever the synergistic erythroid effects of TPO they are dependent on EPO [16,17], and the latter remains the primary regulator of red cell production. Thus, any TPO-induced increase in erythropoiesis would be met by a compensatory decrease in EPO levels, negating any apparent TPO effect on mature red cell production. Therefore, to more fully explore its *in vivo* potential, we next studied whether TPO might augment erythropoiesis in a setting in which EPO levels would not decline, during cytotoxic therapy-induced pancytopenia. Following the administration of sublethal levels of total body irradiation and carboplatinum, the administration of TPO accelerates platelet *and* red cell recovery. The effects on erythropoiesis were marked; 13 days following cytotoxic therapy (the midpoint of control animal recovery) the number of BFU-E had recovered to 20% of normal, CFU-E had rebounded to 60% of normal, and the reticulocyte count was normal in TPO treated mice (16). In contrast, none of three indices of erythropoiesis were detectable in the radiation and chemotherapy vehicle-treated mice. More recent studies using larger animal models have confirmed the effects of TPO on the accelerated recovery of erythroid progenitors [18], but not all investigators have reported favorable effects on mature red cell recovery. At the present it appears that the non-megakaryocytic effects of TPO on haematopoietic recovery may be dependent on the myelosuppressive therapies administered.

TPO affects the survival and proliferation of haematopoietic stem cells

Based on the arguments elaborated in the introductory comments, several investigators have begun to explore whether recombinant TPO exerts effects on primitive haematopoietic cells. Using low concentrations of marrow cells from mice that had been treated two days earlier with 5-fluorouracil and selected for expression of the Sca and c-Kit antigens, Ogawa and colleagues have shown that TPO can act in concert with SCF to augment the number of blast cell colonies which develop, and to induce these primitive progenitors to begin to divide earlier and more often than in the presence of SCF alone [19]. In order to address similar questions, we used a previously published procedure to obtain pure populations of primitive haematopoietic cells. Ten such cells lead to long-term reconstitution of all haematopoietic lineages in 100% of lethally irradiated recipients, but do not contain CFU-S^{d12}, CFU-S^{d8} or any type of mature *in vitro* colony-forming cells. Using single cell cultures we found that by itself TPO supports the survival of a fraction of such cells but not their proliferation [20]. However, when TPO was added to these cultures in the presence of IL-3 or SCF the number of cells which began to divide was greater than that seen in IL-3-only or SCF-only containing cultures, they entered the cell cycle sooner, and the total number of cells and number of committed progenitors of all lineages were far greater [20].

A number of observations suggest that these *in vitro* effects of TPO on the haematopoietic stem cell are manifest *in vivo*. For example, as partly discussed above, the administration of TPO to normal mice augments not only megakaryocytic progenitors but also the number of BFU-E. Moreover, both marrow and splenic granulocyte and monocyte progenitors also increase [21]. However, the most compelling data for an effect of TPO on multiple aspects of haematopoiesis are derived from TPO and Mpl knock-out mice. In both animals the number of all types of mature and primitive progenitor cells (BFU-E, CFU-GM, CFU-MK, CFU-Blast) are reduced to 10-40% of normal values [22,23]. Thus, the *in vitro* effects of TPO on multiple aspects of haematopoiesis are mirrored by its *in vivo* properties.

Thrombopoietin has moved from the theoretical to reality in a few short years. As it now moves to clinical trials we should keep in mind the lessons learned from its *in vitro* properties. The therapeutic effects of TPO may be greater than initially anticipated.

References

1. Kaushansky K. Thrombopoietin: The primary regulator of platelet production. Blood 1995;86:419-31.
2. Lok S, Kaushansky K, Holly RD, et al. Cloning and expression of murine thrombopoietin cDNA and stimulation of platelet production *in vivo*. Nature 1994;369:565-68.
3. Bartley TD, Bogenberger J, Hunt P, et al. Identification and cloning of a megakaryocyte growth and development factor that is a ligand for the cytokine receptor Mpl. Cell 1994;77:1117-24.
4. de Sauvage FJ, Hass PE, Spencer SD, et al. Stimulation of megakaryocytopoiesis and thrombopoiesis by the c-Mpl ligand. Nature 1994;369:533.
5. Vigon I, Mornon J-P, Cocault L, et al. Molecular cloning and characterization of *MPL*, the human homolog of the v-*mpl* oncogene: Identification of a member of the haematopoietic growth factor receptor superfamily. Proc Natl Acad Sci USA 1992;89:5640-44.
6. Wendling F, Varlet P, Charon M, Tambourin P. A retrovirus complex inducing an acute myeloproliferative leukemia disorder in mice. Virology 1986;149:242-46.
7. Vigon I, Dreyfus F, Melle J, et al. Expression of the *c-mpl* proto-oncogene in human haematologic malignancies. Blood 1993;82:877-83.
8. McDonald TP, Sullivan PS. Megakaryocytic and erythrocytic cell lines share a common precursor cell. Exp Haematol 1993;21:1316-20.

9. Hunt P. A bipotential megakaryocyte/erythrocyte progenitor cell: The link between erythropoiesis and megakaryopoiesis becomes stronger. J Lab Clin Med 1995;125: 303-04.
10. Papayannopoulou Th, Brice M, Farrer D, Kaushansky K. Insights into the cellular mechanisms of erythropoietin-thrombopoietin synergy. Exp Haematol 1996;24:660-69.
11. Debili N, Coulombel L, Croisille L, et al. Characterization of a bipotent erythro-megakaryocytic progenitor in human bone marrow. Blood 1996;88:1284-96.
12. Tronik-Le-Roux D, Roullot V, Schweitzer A, Berthier R, Marguerie G: Suppression of erythro-megakaryocytopoiesis and the induction of reversible thrombocytopenia in mice transgenic for the thymidine kinase gene targeted by the platelet glycoprotein alpha lib promoter. J Exp Med 1995;181:2141-51.
13. Broudy VC, Lin NL, Kaushansky K. Thrombopoietin (c-*mpl* ligand) acts synergistically with erythropoietin, stem cell factor, and IL-11 to enhance murine megakaryocyte colony growth and increases megakaryocyte ploidy *in vitro*. Blood 1995;85:1719-26.
14. McDonald TP, Cottrell MB, Clift RE, Cullen WC, Lin FK. High doses of recombinant erythropoietin stimulate platelet production in mice. Exp Haematol 1997;15:719-21.
15. Ikebuchi K, Clark SC, Ihle JN, et al.: Granulocyte colony-stimulating factor enhances interleukin 3-dependent proliferation of multipotential hemopoietic progenitors. Proc Natl Acad Sci USA 1988;85:3445-49.
16. Kaushansky K, Broudy, VC, Grossmann A, et al. Thrombopoietin expands erythroid progenitors, increases red cell production, and enhances erythroid recovery after myelosuppressive therapy. J Clin Invest 1995;96:1683-87.
17. Kobayashi M, Laver JH, Kato T, et al. Recombinant human thrombopoietin (Mpl ligand) enhances proliferation of erythroid progenitors. Blood 1995;86:2494-99.
18. Farese AM, Hunt P, Grab LB, MacVittae TJ. Combined administration of recombinant human megakaryocyte growth and development factor and granulocyte colony-stimulating factor enhances multi-lineage haematopoietic reconstitution in nonhuman primates after radiation induced marrow aplasia. J Clin Invest 1996;97:2145-51.
19. Ku H, Yonemura Y, Kaushansky K, Ogawa M. Thrombopoietin, the ligand for the Mpl receptor, synergizes with steel factor and other early-acting cytokines in supporting proliferation of primitive haematopoietic progenitors of mice. Blood 1996;87:4544-51.
20. Sitnicka E, Lin N, Priestley GV, et al. The effect of thrombopoietin on the proliferation and differentiation of murine haematopoietic stem cells. Blood 1996;87:4998-5005.
21. Kaushansky K, Lin N, Grossmann A, et al. Thrombopoietin expands erythroid granulocyte-macrophage and megakaryocytic progenitor cells in normal and myelosuppressed mice. Exp Haematol 1996;23:265-69.
22. Alexander WS, Roberts AW, Nicola NA, et al. Deficiencies in progenitor cells of multiple haematopoietic lineages and defective megakaryocytopoiesis in mice lacking the thrombopoietin receptor c-Mpl. Blood 1996;87:2162-70.
23. Carver-Moore K, Broxmeyer HE, Luoh SM, et al. Low levels of erythroid and myeloid progenitors in thrombopoietin- and *c-mpl*-deficient mice. Blood 1006;88:803-08.

DISCUSSION

D.R. Rill and P.C. Das – moderators

J. Kadar (Hannover, D): Dr. Heddle, I was very impressed by your own study. I have one question which concerns the control of this randomised study: were you able to detect interleukin, cytokine and chemokine levels in the fresh plasma you are using for the rejuvenation of the platelet concentrate? An other control group could be the usage of the same plasma for the storage as well as for the rejuvenation of the platelets.

N.M. Heddle (Hamilton, C): I will deal with the second issue first. We did not include the control that you mentioned in this study. In a study that we reported in the New England Journal of Medicine we separated the plasma supernatant from the cellular part of the platelet product, reinfused it and showed that the plasma supernatant caused most and the severest reactions to platelets[1]. One of our concerns with the plasma replacement used in the current study was the fact that we were centrifuging 5 day old platelets, and that this process could actually harm the platelets and affect their function or viability. To assess this we looked at the 24 hour post transfusion platelet recovery and corrected count increments and there was no difference between the two treatment groups. Therefore, we do not think that manipulating the platelet product is a problem. In terms of cytokine measurements on the plasma that was added to the platelets, we measured the concentration of IL-6 after the plasma had been added to the centrifuged platelet product. Our previous experience with measuring cytokines in fresh frozen plasma shows that the concentrations are very low.

J. Kadar: A brief comment; The manipulation itself could be responsible for the lack of difference between the two groups in term of frequency and side effects, because you are centrifuging the platelets.

N.M. Heddle: There was a significant difference in the frequency and severity of the reactions between the two treatment groups. The results clearly show that manipulating the platelets by removing the old plasma and adding fresh frozen

1. Heddle NM, Klama L, Singer J et al., The role of plasma from platelet concentrates in transfusion reactions. N Engl J Med 1994;33:625-28.

plasma results in a lower frequency of reactions. This is probably due to lower cytokine levels in the manipulated product.

C.Th. Smit Sibinga (Groningen, NL): Dr. Drayer, there is definitely a difference between the approach you showed and the principle presented by dr. Mertelsmann in that you used the patient's own tumour cells to be genetically engineered and given back as a vaccine, where Dr. Mertelsmann is trying to approach the problem through fibrocytes or fibroblasts. Does this have an effect on the duration of the therapy. Would it be possible in your approach to boost after some 4 to 6 months, because you said that by about 5 months time there is a need to revaccinate. Is that necessary and is that possible?

J. I. Drayer (Alameda, CA, USA): I think what we have here is a first development, a first formulation approach to immune treatment in cancer. We have chosen to use the patient's own tumour cells and not fibroblasts, based on preclinical information that at least with GM-CSF in our models we could not prove that having fibroblasts and non-altered tumour cells together would be better than the tumour cells by themselves. But that is just one way of looking at it. It makes it more complex, because dr. Mertelsmann has his fibroblasts ready in storage and he needs very little manipulation with the tumour cells. We need more manipulation and we need a little more time, but that can be overcome. I think the most important aspect right now is that we do have something that has a tendency to work, let us then move with that and later worry about other aspects. What I should say is that transduction of the used tumour cells using retroviral and other vectors is not a problem anymore. GM-CSF secretion is not a problem anymore. Right now we can produce for melanoma for instance vaccines in 90% of patients within 4 to 6 weeks of time. If the testing becomes a little easier, because everyone gets more comfortable with retroviral products and we do not have to do replication competent retroviral testing anymore, it could be ready even within 4 weeks. So, I think methodology will improve and then later the reality will tell us whether more fancy approaches that are immediately available will be as good as what we have shown right now for the crude product as you would say, the patient's own tumour cells.

R.E.M. Toes (Leiden, NL): Maybe in relation to the last question there is now increasing evidence that T-cells are not induced by the tumour cells themselves but rather by lymphoid cells that pick up tumour antigens and then present them to T-cells. Did you consider to use allogeneic tumour cells for your GM-CSF transduction?

J.I. Drayer: I think the argument can go both ways. If you believe that most of the significant antigens were present in the patient's own tumour, taken up by the antigen presenting cells and brought to the immune system with the help of the cytokine, then you could say the patient's own tumour is the best you can give. It is a rarity to find in an allogeneic prepared mix exactly the same antigens that that patient would have. If you look at the data that for instance Don Morton has at the

John Wayne's Cancer Institute in Santa Monica you will find that he has treated over 6,000 patients[1]. He has never seen the kind of a density of an infiltrate that we see. He also has not seen the kind of consistency that we see. He sees some responses which you would anticipate but apparently the degree and the intensity of the response may be less than the methodology that Dr. Mertelsmann is using or that we are using. Prove is not there, there is a need for a direct comparison of these two technologies and the treatment of some of the tumours that we know best and maybe even with other immune products. But at least these are the thoughts that you can go by.

C.Th. Smit Sibinga: Prof. Mulder, do you see a future for a combination of the Groningen approach with the intense ablative cancer chemotherapy and the rescue through CD34 positive cells and a vaccine to sweep out the last amount of tumour by this approach?

N.H. Mulder (Groningen, NL): That would be a very interesting approach, provided you can find some proof of the clinical activity of immune therapy that will emerge in the coming years. Quite another approach may be the experiments from Dr. Vogelzang and others of the United States who induce graft versus host disease after autologous bone marrow transplantation by using lymphokine growth factors and he claims also tumour infiltrates[2]. That might be interesting as we know that in allogeneic bone marrow transplantation graft versus leukaemia has an antitumour effect.

C.Th. Smit Sibinga: Right, so maybe we could further bridge and narrow the gap.

N.H. Mulder: Hopefully, yes.

B. Löwenberg (Rotterdam, NL): Dr. Dale, you postulated the hypothesis that patients with severe infections, with pneumonias would raise perhaps a suboptimal granulocyte response, and this was the basis for the rationale of the study. Although the granulocytic response was not maximal, it was probably adequate in most patients, because you could not improve outcome. My question is, what is the future. Would there be a place for granulocyte transfusions then, if the *in vivo* response in most patients is adequate?

My second question is: are there prognostic factors that allow you to prospectively identify those patients, that may raise a suboptimal response and would perhaps benefit from granulocytes or G-CSF treatment *in vivo*?

1. Morton DL, Barth A. Vaccine therapy for malignant melanoma. CA Cancer J Clin 1996; 46:225-44.
2. Kennedy MJ, Hess AD, Passos Coelho J-L et al. Cyclosporine A (CsA) induces autologous graft vs host disease (AGVHD) following high dose chemotherapy (HDC) supported with peripheral blood progenitor cell (PBPC) infusions alone. Proc ASCO 1996;15:abstract 964.

D.C. Dale (Seattle, WA, USA): I think we have come to accept that neutrophils are important in the acute response to infection and the consequences of not having enough neutrophils are well known to us. But just how many are needed for the optimal response is not known and I think that is the kind of issue that a study like this raises. In some recent work in Seattle[1,2] we have found that in fact people who are severely neutropenic, neutrophil transfusions appear to be a benefit.The benefit of raising the neutrophil counts in antibiotic-treated patients with acute infections and normal haematopiesis is still open. The data I showed suggest that for the sickest patients accentuating the neutrophil response maybe helpful. One of the reasons why that is of such interest at this time is the problem around the world of the emergence of antibiotic-resisting organisms, and not just in tuberculosis but also in pneumococcal and staphylococcal and enterococcal infections. Among common organisms there is a gradual but very important emergence of resistance and that is one of the reasons for being interested in new ways to enhance the host response.

B. Löwenberg: Are you able to identify those patients prior to treatment?

D.C. Dale: Yes, I think in some ways. For instance, in the study I showed, the patients with multi-lobal pneumonia could have been identified at admission in the hospital. If low blood pressure is a marker, which I believe it may be, that will be useful. The third clinical criterium I suspect will be important, will be a low white blood cell count or neutrophil count at admission to a hospital. But these are only predictions; more research is needed to identify and validate predictors of benefit.

C.Th. Smit Sibinga: Dr. Toes, what I would like to know is what is actually the procedure. How did you isolate the dendritic cells and how sure were you that you had a pure population of dendritic cells before starting to manipulate them?

R.E.M. Toes: The isolation is relatively simple. We just take the bone marrow of mice and culture these bone marrow cells for 8 days in the presence of GM-CSF and IL-4. When we analyse the cells on FacsScan there are dendritic cells present as we can identify them by monoclonal antibodies. There are also many other cells present. But we think dendritic cells are doing the trick, because when we isolate splenic dendritic cells, a rather homologous dendritic cell population, we also induce tumour-protective immunity. The same cannot be induced when we load the peptides on for example spleen cells. So, it is actually a functional definition; we call it a dendritic cell, but we are not completely sure.

---

1. Maakestad K, Mazanet R, Liles WC, Dale DC. Neutrophil transfusions for treatment of infections. In: Morstyn G, Sheridan WP eds. Cell Therapy 1st ed. Cambridge University Press, Cambridge, UK 1996:510-26.
2. Dale DC, Liles WC, Llewellyn C, Roger E, Bowden R, Price TH. Neutrophil transfusion therapy: characteristics and kinetics of cells from donors treated with a combination of G-CSF and dexamethasone. Blood 1996:88(Suppl):627a.

C.Th. Smit Sibinga: With regard to the tumour vaccine approach we have now heard three variants of approaches. The variant of Mertelsmann, of Drayer using the autologous tumour cells, and your mouse model variant on dendritic cells. Do you think that each of these approaches may be used for specific tumours, or do you think that they might be applicable for the whole range of solid tumours?

R.E.M. Toes: Well in the case of dendritic cells, you have to load them with tumour derived peptides, or tumour antigens and in that case it will only be applicable for a certain type of tumour. But the same is true for when you go for an autologous tumour vaccine. Maybe not when you have a fibroblast vector transfected with different tumour antigens or with different cytokines, then you may achieve a broader range of tumours that can be treated. But for dendritic cells you have to administer the peptide antigens as a protein or as a gene or as a peptide to the dendritic cell and then you are really focusing on one type of tumour, but you are also focusing on a defined specificity that only attacks tumours, so that is the advantage.

C.Th. Smit Sibinga: Dr. Kaushansky, earlier in the meeting we spoke about the propagation of cells, the culturing of stem cells bringing them into multiplication for which cocktails of cytokines are used. Do you think that, if we now have thrombopoietin as a dominant lineage substance, that that could replace part of the other cytokines and growth factors in the cocktails?

K. Kaushansky (Seattle, WA, USA): That is a difficult question to answer. We have limited data; another group has looked at varying combinations of cytokines. I would expect, if your goal is to expand all lineages of cells, that adding thrombopoietin would probably be a good idea. Several groups have now clearly demonstrated important effects of thrombopoietin on primitive cells and on various types of intermediate progenitor cells, making it likely to exert some benefit in an *ex vivo* expansion system. The question of whether it actually finds clinical utility will be dictated by more political/economic reasons! There is not a lot of cooperation between some of the biotech companies, what actually turns out to be the cytokine cocktail used in *ex vivo* expansion trials in people may not necessarily be based on a whole spectrum of cytokines. Speaking purely scientifically I expect it would be of some advantage.

N. Choudhury (Lucknow, Ind): Dr. Kaushansky, I was very much impressed by your presentation. It is just curiosity; what is the future of thrombopoietin in clinical transfusion medicine. Can we use it for stimulation of donors and collection of platelets or some clinical application?

K. Kaushansky: It is clear that treatment of platelet donors is a major area of clinical interest. I just attended a meeting a short time ago at the National Institute of Health in the US, where we discussed some of the clinical aspects of thrombopoietin. Time and again the application of thrombo-poietin as a way to improve the efficiency to obtain platelet donations was raised. There is still a lingering concern over safety; there is data to suggest that when you raise the platelet count in a normal animal you see more deposition of platelets on a thrombogenic surface. It is not disproportionate; if you have a platelet count that is 5 times greater, you see about 5 times more platelets laid down on a thrombogenic surface. However, the platelets being produced in thrombopoietin-stimulated normal people are normal platelets. We have seen reactive thrombocytosis patients with a million platelets who have absolutely no problem whatsoever; even 2 million platelets. So, I suspect that in the realm of transfusion medicine administering just one dose or at most two doses to a donor, you will easily be able to harvest 4 to 5 times as many platelets. Whether thrombopoietin is applied to *ex vivo* expansion to harvest platelets might be a more difficult question. The reason is that although suspension cultures grown with thrombopoietin will yield platelets, the process is not efficient. It is not clear if that is correctable in culture or whether it is going to require some sort of stromal interaction. In the bone marrow megakaryocytes grow next to endothelial cells and it may be that they are providing some important signals for actually making platelets. I think it is clear that thrombopoietin will find a role in expanding platelets for transfusion, whether it finds itself in the role of growing platelets in the test tube, or in a bag is uncertain.

N. Choudhury: The theme of the symposium is cytokines and growth factors in blood transfusion, so in presence of erythropoietin, thrombopoietin and what may be the future of artificial blood.

K. Kaushansky: Well, clearly from my point of view the most important of these is thrombopoietin.

R. Coelho (Lisbon, Port): Dr. Toes, when you administer the peptide to animals, do you usually get CD34 positive CTL's, because it is an exogenous peptide or do you get more CTL lines?

R.E.M. Toes: Well, we immunise with peptides that only represent CTL epitopes; so when we immunise with these peptides we get CTL responses as is the case in the HPV 16 system. In the case of the adeno system, we only deplete adeno-specific CD8 responses. We do not measure CD4, so I do not think they are there.

H.J.C. de Wit (Leeuwarden, NL): Dr. Heddle, you showed in concordance with the results of Dr. Muylle, that blood products in particular platelet concentrates stored with leukocytes produce cytokines that can generate transfusion reactions. We have been focused on producing leukocyte poor products. On the other hand there have been developments in platelet storage solutions of which the problem was that long term storage was quite difficult to achieve. Would it be a reasonable approach to spin off the plasma and replace by a simple storage solution 2-3 hours before transfusion and avoid expensive filters, or expensive storage solutions?

N.M. Heddle: Yes, that certainly would be feasible, but I do not think that you even need to use these storage solutions, you can just concentrate the platelets. The only reason that we added fresh frozen plasma back onto the platelets as a replacement, was to keep the study blind, so that the two products looked identical. This was important because the outcome measure was very subjective. What we are routinely using now is sort of a step-wise approach. If a patient has two reactions all we do is concentrate the platelets. We spin them down and we remove all of the plasma except for about 50 ml. The product is transfused in that form. If a patient then goes on to have two additional reactions to the plasma depleted platelets, we will then leukodeplete. We have had a few patients that have required plasma removal plus leukoreduction, but so far none of the patients that are given both interventions have had reactions necessitating a third approach. The approach that we would use is probably a combination of fresh single donor platelets and perhaps additional premedication..

B. Löwenberg: You eliminated a significant proportion of the transfusion reactions by removing plasma, but still dealt with a significant percentage of transfusion reactions in these patients. That was quite notable. What is your explanation? Could these perhaps be alloimmunisation reactions, because your patients had already a history of transfusion. Or is there another explanation?

N.M. Heddle: That is a good question. Certainly when we designed the study, we expected that we would go from about a 25% reaction rate and estimated a 50% reduction to 12 or 13 percent. I was a little surprised, that it was as high as 17% although the reactions that did occur with the plasma replacement were very mild. One could question how clinically significant these reactions really were. What caused those reactions? Certainly our New England Journal publication[1] suggested that there are at least two mechanisms, because some patients in that study only reacted to the cellular component. So, I think the antibody mediated mechanism, which I personally feel as the predominant mechanism for red cell reactions, probably does contribute to some platelet reactions. With platelet transfusions biological response modifiers (cytokines), are the predominant cause of reactions. But if you look at the apheresis platelets collected by the Cobe Spectra that are prestorage leukoreduced and have less than 10^6 leukocytes, you still have a 2 or 3 percent reaction rate. So, I suspect that there is another mechanism, which we have not identified yet.

C. Marsman (Leeuwarden, NL): Dr. Heddle, you showed apheresis thrombocyte concentrates having much lower levels of interleukines and other cytokines compared to pooled platelet concentrate. Might there be a relation or an interaction between the leukocytes of the various donors. Could it be that the less donors you use the less cytokines you might find?

---

1. Heddle NM, Klama L, Singer J et al., The role of plasma from platelet concentrates in transfusion reactions. N Engl J Med 1994;33:625-28.

N.M. Heddle: That is an interesting question and I really do not know the answer. We have done some preliminary studies where we pooled several platelet concentrates prepared by the PRP technique that we use in North America and measured cytokines. Pooling did not show any increase in cytokines. I think that observation is consistent with the buffy coat method, that is used in parts of Europe, where buffy coats are pooled together to make the platelets. It is my understanding that cytokine levels do not increase in those products. So, I do not know the answer to your question, but I think that the preliminary information that we have suggests that pooling probably is not an issue; however, it does need to be studied further.

T.L. Goodnough (St. Louis, MO, USA): Dr. Heddle, I do not remember if you showed us IL-6 levels, for example in stored red cell units.

N.M. Heddle: Yes, actually IL-6 is not detectable in either buffy coat depleted red cells or in the red cells prepared after platelet rich plasma was removed. You do detect low levels of IL-1. We just recently did the comparison of those two types of products. Another interesting observation which will be presented at the AABB[1] is IL-8 data. With the buffy coat red cells we detected IL-8 on day 1 of storage. The levels were much lower than those found in platelets. Over 42 days of storage IL-8 levels decreased. I am not an expert on IL-8, but it is my understanding that IL-8 can be absorbed to red cells and that may actually be what is accounting for the decrease. It certainly looks like the method of producing red cells from a buffy coat technique generates slightly more IL-8 than red cells produced by the PRP method. The low levels of cytokines in red cell products makes me think that the red cell reactions are probably predominantly antibody mediated as opposed to cytokine mediated.

B. Löwenberg: Dr. Kaushansky, as far as the effects of TPO are concerned on other lineages, how did you examine TPO receptor expression in subpopulations of progenitor cells? How sure are you that these effects of TPO are direct and not indirect?

K. Kaushansky: On the stem cells that I showed you we have performed RTPCR on as few as 20 cells and find a clear signal. We have not yet done the experiment on one cell, but as far as we know these are homogeneous cells. For BFU-E there are two papers; one from our group[2] and from Makio Ogawa's group[3], which was more elegant. They plucked individual BFU-E colonies after 4 days at the 4 and 8

---

1. Heddle NM, Klama L, Meyer R et al. A comparison of two interventions to prevent platelet reactions. Transfusion 1996;36:47S.
2. Kaushansky K, Broudy VC, Grossmann A et al. Thrombopoietin expands erythroid progenitors, increases red cell production, and enhances erythroid recovery after myelosuppressive therapy. J Clin Invest 1995;96:1683-87.
3. Kobayashi M, Laver JH, Kato T et al. Recombinant human thrombopoietin (Mpl ligand) enhances proliferation of erythroid progenitors. Blood 1995;86:2494-99.

cell level and then washed them free of growth factors and plated them in a secondary culture. So all they were picking were BFU-E progeny from the culture and then growing them in the presence of erythropoietin with or without thrombopoietin. Doing that experiment, which is quite a pure population of cells you see a threefold increase in the number of BFU-E colonies that develop from that population of cells, in the presence of thrombopoietin than in its absence. The stem cells that we are culturing are single cells. From all of those criteria we believe that the effect of thrombopoietin is direct.

IV. FUTURE POTENTIAL OF CYTOKINES AND GROWTH FACTORS IN TRANSFUSION MEDICINE

ERYTROPOIETIN – WHERE DO WE GO FROM HERE?

L.T. Goodnough

Introduction

Despite significant reduction in blood risks [1], practice guidelines have recommended the development of alternatives to blood [2-4]. It has been nearly 10 years since the initial demonstration of the efficacy of recombinant human erytropoietin (EPO) therapy to correct the anaemia of chronic renal failure [5]. EPO therapy has also been approved for the treatment of the anaemia of chronic renal insufficiency, the anaemia of cancer and cancer therapy, and the aenimia of human immunodeficiency virus (HIV) positive patients undergoing azovudine therapy [6]. Additionally, EPO therapy has been approved for use in conjunction with autologous blood procurement in Australia since 1992 and in Europe since 1994. The Circular of Information for the Use of Human Blood and Blood Components, issued jointly by the American Red Cross, the Council of Community Blood Centers and the American Association of Blood Banks, includes EPO (along with iron, vitamin B_{12}, and folic acid) as a specific medication that should be used instead of blood transfusion "if the clinical condition of the patient permits sufficient time for these agents to promote erythropoiesis" [7]. A number of clinical trials that have studied the role of EPO therapy as an alternative to allogeneic blood transfusion in the perisurgical period have now been completed. The pertinent clinical studies of EPO in each of these areas are reviewed, to provide a framework for clinicians in the use of EPO in patients undergoing surgical procedures associated with blood loss-induced anaemia.

Facilitation of autologous blood predeposit

Recent publications have emphasized that when elective decision to transfuse is made, the preferred alternative is autologous blood [4]. This previously under-utilized practice [8] has now become a standard of care in certain elective surgical procedures [9,10], and there has been a significant increase in the percentage of blood collected nationally that is autologous [11]. The relationship between the ordering of autologous blood, its collection, and subsequent exposure to allogeneic blood was examined in a recent study of 263 orthopaedic surgical patients [12]. Eightyfour (32%) of 263 patients were unable to store the number of autologous blood units requested, of which 70 (83%) were female patients. Only 3 (2%) of 147 patients asked to donate ≤ 3 units received autologous blood, compared to 20 (17%)

of 116 patients asked to donate ≥4 units (P<0.01). The most important determinant for the risk of subsequent allogeneic blood transfusion has been identified to be the presence of anaemia at first blood donation, especially in patients asked to pre-donate ≥4 autologous units [12].

Studies of endogenous erythropoietin levels in allogeneic blood donors further suggested that treatment with EPO might correct or prevent the development of anaemia in these pateints during blood donation, and increase the volume of autologous blood that could be collected before surgery [13,14]. This was demonstrated in a randomized, placebo-controlled, study in which non-anaemic patients who received EPO twice weekly (600 u/kg intravenously) were able to donate 41% more red blood cell volume than placebo-treated patients [15]. A subsequent analysis [16] of preoperative red blood cell production (taking into account both *in vivo* and *ex vivo* (stored) red blood cell volumes) in the placebo patients who underwent aggressive autologous blood phlebotomy (procurement of six units beginning 25-35 days before surgery) demonstrated a significant (27%) expansion of red blood cell volume over a four week period. However, the 47% RBC volume expansion observed in the EPO-treated patients was statistically greater, resulting in the generation of nearly five blood units preoperatively compared to three blood units for the placebo-treated patients. The major difference in red blood cell expansion between the placebo-treated and EPO-treated groups occurred early in the collection period; by the time of surgery, the endogenous erythropoietin effect in the placebo-treated patients diminished the differences between groups. Two subsequent clinical trials have demonstrated that among non-anaemia patients who undergo orthopedic procedures, no clinical benefit is seen if EPO (150 u/kg to 600 u/kg intravenously for six doses over three weeks) is administered during the donation period [17,18]. A third trial [19] of subcutaneous EPO (500 u/kg delivered in six doses over three weeks) in 95 patients undergoing joint replacement surgery demonstrated lower allogeneic blood exposure in EPO-treated patients compared to placebo-treated patients in the control group (10% vs 35%, respectively). In this study, however, patients were asked to predonate only two autologous blood units, which may have contributed to the relatively high allogeneic blood exposure rate in the placebo-treated group. For non-anaemic pateints, autologous blood phlebotomy for liquid blood storage (35-42 days) remains an alternative to EPO therapy if they can tolerate aggressive blood donation and achieve the resultant stimulation of endogenous erythropoietin.

A subsequent European clinical trial in anaemic (Hct ≤40%) orthopaedic patients asked to predonate ≥4 autologous units reported that EPO therapy reduced allogeneic blood transfusion during surgery when compared to placebo-treated patients [20]. However, this result was achieved only with intravenously administered supplemental iron. A second United States multi-center trial in orthopaedic patients who were anaemic (HCT ≤39%) at first donation also evaluated EPO therapy (with oral supplemental iron) during aggressive autologous blood phlebotomy. This study found that 20% of the EPO-treated patients (600 u/kg intravenously for six doses) subsequently had allogeneic blood transfusion, compared to 31% of the placebo-treated patients [21]. While the difference did not reach statistical significance, this and the previously-cited trial [20] domonstrate that diminished allogeneic exposure is possible in anaemic patients who are treated with both EPO and iron therapy, compared to those receiving iron therapy alone.

Enhancement of haemodilution

Acute isovolemic haemodilution entails the removal of blood from a patient shortly before an anticipated significant surgical blood loss, while restoring the circulating blood volume with acellular fluid. The rationale for the use of haemodilution is that it is beter to lose blood at a lower rather than a higher level of haematocrit. With haemodilution, the number of units to be withdrawn depends on the expected replacement needs, the initial haematocrit, and the minimum level of haematocrit the patient can safely tolerate. It has been recommended to remove blood until the haematocrit is at a certain value e.g., 27-30% under conditions of "moderate" haemodilution [22]. Recently the efficacy of haemodilution to this range of haematocrit has been questioned [23,24]. The removal of three blood units in a 100 kg man with a reduction of preoperative haematocrit level from 44% to 32% and who subsequently undergoes radical prostatectomy with an estimated blood loss of 2600 ml, results in 732 ml in RBC lost. This can be compared to 947 ml RBC that would have been lost if haemodilution had not been performed. Thus, the surgical RBC volume loss "saved" by haemodilution in this patient represents only 215 ml, or the equivalent of approximately one blood unit [25].

Nevertheless, a recent controlled study concluded that moderate haemodilution is a cost-effective alternative to autologous blood predeposit in patients undergoing radical prostatectomy [26]. Thirty consecutive patients were analyzed and compared to 30 retrospective, matched control patients who had undergone radical prostatectomy without haemodilution; these thirty control patient had each predonated three autologous blood units. Both groups had three (10%) patients who received allogeneic blood transfusion, yet the total costs calculated for blood conservation and blood transfusion were 30% lower in the patients who had undergone acute haemodilution compared to those patients who had predonated autologous blood.

One approach to enhancing the safety and efficacy of haemodilution is to couple the technique with EPO therapy. Recently, moderate haemodilution (up to four units or to a haematocrit level of 28%), with or without EPO therapy (given at 600 u/kg subcutaneously at three weeks and two weeks before surgery, and at 300 u/kg on the day of surgery), was compared to the preoperative autologous donation of three units in patients undergoing radical prostatectomy [27]. This study found that preoperative EPO therapy was effective in minimizing the perioperative anaemia associated with haemodilution and surgical blood loss; the mean nadir haematocrit level exceeded 30% throughout the surgical hospitalization. The preservation of red cell volume resulted in the transfusion of only one allogeneic blood unit to one of 24 patients in the EPO-treated group. This represented a substantial improvement over haemodilution alone (six of 26 patients transfused with 16 allogeneic units) or preoperative autologous donation alone (four of 26 patients transfused with five allogeneic units).

Stimulation of erythropoiesis

With the recent recognition that autologous blood donation is poorly cost-effective [10,26,28,29] several clinical trials have evaluated EPO therapy in surgical patients who did not undergo autologous blood procurement. In a multicenter Canadian study [30] of 208 patients undergoing elective primary or revision hip athroplasty, group I (78 patients) received 14 days of placebo, group II (77 patients) received 14 days of subcutaneous EPO (300 u/kg) beginning 10 days before surgery and group III (53 patients) received 9 days of EPO (300 u/kg) beginning 5 days before surgery. Twentyfour percent of patients in group II and 29% of patients in group III received blood transfusion rates significantly less than in 42% patients who were treated with placebo. However, thirty (45%) group III patients also received transfusions, indicating that EPO therapy initiated within five days of surgery is not effective in preventing allogeneic blood exposure. A multicenter study of 200 patients undergoing orthopaedic surgery in the United States [31] has also been conducted, in which 54 patients were treated with subcutaneous EPO (300 u/kg) for 15 days, beginning 10 days before surgery; 64 patients were treated with EPO at a lower dose (100 u/kg); and 67 patients received placebo. In this study, 36 (54%) of the placebo patients were transfused, significantly greater than 16 (25%) of the lower (100 u/kg) EPO dose group and 9 (17%) of the higher (300 u/kg) EPO dose group. These two studies demonstrate that EPO therapy is effective as a pharmacologic alternative to allogeneic blood in elective orthopaedic surgical patients who do not have autologous blood available. A follow-up study demonstrated that four weekly doses of 600 u/kg was comparable to a daily dose of 300 u/kg over 15 days [32].

In summary, recombinant human erythropoietin therapy has been shown to be an affective alternative to red cell transfusion in patients undergoing surgical procedures. There are a number of clinical settings where EPO therapy has been demonstrated to reduce allogeneic blood exposure. The challenge for surgeons, anaesthesiologists and transfusion medicine specialists will be to combine the use of this biotechnology product, along with other conservation strategies, so that it becomes safer and at least cost-equivalent to allogeneic red cell therapy in the surgical setting.

References

1. Lackritz EM, Satten GA, Aberle-Grasse J, et al. Estimated risk of transmission of the human immunodeficiency virus by screened blood in the United States. N Engl J Med 1995;333:1721-25.
2. Skolnick AA. As the blood supply gets safer, experts still call for ways to reduce the need for transfusions. JAMA 1992;268:698-700.
3. Welch HG, Meehan KR, Goodnough LT. Prudent strategies for elective red blood cell

transfusion. Ann Intern Med 1992;116:393-406.
4. American College of Physicians. Practice strategies for elective red blood cell transfusion. Ann Int Med 1992;115:403-06.
5. Eschbach JW, Egrie JC, Downing MR, Browne JK, Adamson JW. Correction of the anaemia of end stage renal disease with recombinant human erythropoietin: Results of a combined phase I and phase II clinical trial. N Engl J Med 1987;316:73-78.
6. Goodnough LT, Anderson KC, Kurtz S, et al. Indications and guidelines for the use of haematopoietic growth factors. Transfusion 1993;33:944-59.
7. Circular of Information for the Use of Human Blood Components. Joint Council of the American Red Cross, Council of Community Blood Centers, and American Association of Blood Banks. March 1994:p6.
8. Toy PTCY, Strauss R, Stehling L, et al. Predeposit autologous blood for elective surgery: A multicenter study. N Engl J Med 1987:316:517-20.
9. Goodnough LT, Shafron D, Marcus RE. Impact of preoperative autologous blood donation in elective orthopaedic surgery. Vox Sang 1990;59:65-69.
10. Goodnough LT, Grishaber JE, Birkmeyer JD, Monk TG, Catalona WJ. Efficacy and cost-effectiveness of autologous blood predeposit in patients undergoing radical prostatectomy procedures. Urology 1994;44:226-31.
11. Wallace EL, Churchill WH, Surgenor DM, et al. Collection and transfusion of blood and blood components in the United States, 1992. Transfusion 1995;35:802-12.
12. Goodnough LT, Vizmeg, Robecks R, Schwartz A, Soegiarso W. Prevalence and classification of anaemia in elective orthpaedic surgery patients: Implications for blood conservation program. Vox Sang 1992;63:90-95.
13. Goodnough LT, Brittenham G. Limitations of the erythropoietic response to serial phlebotomy: Implications of autologous blood donor programs. J Lab Clin Med 1990; 115:28-35.
14. Kickler TS, Spivak JL. Effect of repeated whole blood donations on serum immunoreactive erythropoietin levels in autologous donors. JAMA 1988;260:65-67.
15. Goodnough LT, Rudick S, Price TH, et al. Increased collection of autologous blood preoperatively with recombinant human erythropoietin therapy. N Engl J Med 1989; 321:1163-67.
16. Goodnough LT, Price TH, Rudnick S. Preoperative red blood cell production in patients undergoing aggressive autologous blood phlebotomy with and without erythropoietin therapy. Transfusion 1992;32:441-45.
17. Goodnough LT, Price TH and the EPO Study Group. A phase III trial recombinant human erythropoietin therapy in non-anaemic orthopaedic patients subjected to aggressive autologous blood phlebotomy: Dose, response, toxicity, and efficacy. Transfusion 1994;34:66-71.
18. Beris P, Mermillod B, Levy G, et al. Recombinant human erythropoietin as adjuvant treatment for autologous blood donation. Vox Sang 1993;65:212-18.
19. Biesma DH, Marx JJ, Kraaijenhagen RJ, Franke W, Messinger D, Van de Wiel A. Lower homologous blood requirement in autologous blood donors after treatment with recombinant human erythropoietin. Lancet 1994;344:367-70.
20. Mercuriali F, Zanella A, Barosi G, et al. Use erythropoietin to increase the volume of autologous blood donated by orthopaedic patients. Transfusion 1993;33:55-59.
21. Price TH, Goudnough LT, Vogler W, et al. The effect of recombinant erythropoietin administration on the efficacy of autologous blood donation in patients with low haematocrits. Transfusion 1996;36:29-36.
22. Messmer K, Kreimeier M, Intagliett A. Present state of intentional haemodilution. Eur Surg Res 1986;18:254-63.
23. Goodnough LT, Grishaber J, Monk TG, Catalona WJ. Acute preoperative haemo-

dilution in patients undergoing radical prostatectomy: A case study analysis of efficacy. Anesth Analg 1994;78:932-37.
24. Brecher ME, Rosenfeld. Mathematical and computer modelling of acute normovolemic haemodilution. Transfusion 1994;34:176-79.
25. Goodnough LT, Bravo J, Hsueh Y, Keating L, Brittenham GM. Red blood cell volume in autologous and homologous units: Implications of risk/benefit assessment for autologous blood "crossover" and directed blood transfusion. Transfusion 1989;29:821-22.
26. Monk TG, Goodnough LT, Birkmeyer JD, Brecher ME, Catalona WJ. Acute normovolemic hemodilution is a cost-effective alternative to preoperative autologous donation in patients undergoing radical retropubic prostatectomy. Transfusion 1995;35: 559-65.
27. Monk TG, Goodnough LT, Andriole GL, Colberg JW, Lemon DJ, Martin. Preoperative recombinant human erythropoietin therapy enhances the efficacy of acute normovolemic hemodilution. Anest Analg 1995;80:S320.
28. Etchason J, Petz L, Keeler, et al. Cost-effectiveness of autologous blood donation. N Engl J Med 1995;332:719-24.
29. Birkmeyer JD, Goodnough LT, AuBuchon JP, Noordsy PG, Littenberg B. The cost-effectiveness of preoperative autologous blood donation for total hip and knee replacement. Transfusion 1994;34:501-06.
30. Canadian Orthopedic Perioperative Erythropoietin Study Group. Effectiveness of perioperative recombinant human erythropoietin in elective hip replacement. Lancet 1993;341:1227-32.
31. Faris PM, Ritter MA, Abels RI. The effects of recombinant human erythropoietin on perioperative transfusion requirements in patients undergoing major orthopaedic surgery. J Bone J Surg 1996;78A:62-72.
32. Goldberg MA, McCutchen JW, Jove M, et al. A safety and efficacy comparison study of two dosing regimens of erythropoietin alpha in patients undergoing major orthopedic surgery. Amer J Ortho 1996;258:544-52.

ETHICAL ASPECTS OF THE USE OF CYTOKINES AND GROWTH FACTORS IN DONORS

H.M. Dupuis

Introduction

The altruistic practice of blood donation by healthy donors has gradually become more common. Apart from the matter of payment, it has never raised many ethical questions. The problems involved are almost exclusively technical and usually relate to possible risks for patients requiring transfusions. Recipients of blood donations have contracted severe contagions through viruses. HIV, for example, has been transmitted to many hemophilia patients. While these are tragic occasions of unforeseen disaster, the moral principles and values involved are not subject to debate. Over the last ten to fifteen years, however, the matter of possible harm to donors has developed into a moral dilemma. The issue raised is whether harming or creating risks for healthy, volunteer donors can ever be justified.

An uncomfortable case

The following incident occurred recently in a Dutch hospital. A patient with a severe and recurring leukemia developed an immediate need for a stem cell transfusion. His team of physicians debated whether it would be justifiable to ask his brother to donate as the procedure would involve growth-factor stimulation. Eventually the brother was approached and agreed to participate. One could ask, "what other choice did he have?"

The experts who were consulted, however, expressed serious doubts and were reluctant to give their consent. They were concerned that the team was unable to provide adequate information on possible harmful side-effects to the donor. Nevertheless, despite these concerns, and in light of the life-threatening situation of the patient, the procedure was initiated. within twenty-four hours the patient died from the leukemia and the donation never took place. Despite the fact that the patient's prognosis had already been deemed hopeless, his brother was unnecessarily subjected to the stimulation procedure.

This is exemplary of the lack of wisdom and deficient reasoning which periodically accompanies medical decisions and procedures. One wonders how this team of physicians rationalized soliciting the cooperation of the brother in order to facilitate the treatment of a patient who was already near death and for whom treatment was apparently too late. Where was their concern for the consenting brother's health?

While it is easy to raise these questions afterwards, it remains difficult to accept that the medical team was entirely unaware of the gravity of the patient's condition. Still, they did not hesitate to jeopardize the health of the donor or at least expose him to uncertain risks.

"Where is the wisdom.... ?"[1]

This title of a 1991 editorial by British Medical Journal editor Richard Smith, is taken from a quotation by T.S. Eliot: "Where is the wisdom we have lost in knowledge, and where is the knowledge we have lost in information?" Smith quotes Eliot with the intention of emphasizing the general problem of irrationality in medicine. He notes that according to David Eddy, only 15% of all medical intervention is supported by solid scientific evidence – a percentage cited three years earlier by Kerr L. White, director of the prestigious Rockefeller Foundation [2]. According to Smith and Eddy, this may be explained in part "... because only 1% of the articles in medical journals are scientifically sound and partly because many treatments have never been assessed at all." Obviously doctors are not particularly scrupulous when it comes to their own conduct, acting on the basis of non-existing or weak evidence. And as these criticisms stem from physicians themselves there is no reason to doubt their accuracy. Statistics and sound figures do not play the role in medical practice that one would expect.

It seems clear that insufficient knowledge continues to beset modern medicine. Yet at the same time a certain eagerness to treat can be observed among many physicians. Obviously this often noted eagerness is not grounded in reliable research. As such, there must be other explanations. Perhaps it may be attributed to psychological needs on the part of both doctors and patients, doctors feeling compelled to act and patients seeking assistance. Morally, as Lynn Payer so aptly observes, there appears to be confusion between "doing something" and "accomplishing something" [3]. More to the point, many physicians mistakenly equate "doing something" with "doing well".

Indeed, there is something wrong with this identification of activity as beneficence. Medical interventions are often harmful in their own right. Therefore, only a reasonable expectation that something valuable for the patient will ensue can justify the introduction of treatment(s) bearing negative side-effects. In the case of patients with life-threatening conditions, it is widely accepted that physicians may initiate novel and experimental treatments, within reason. Clearly, irrational treatment should never take place, even if life itself is at stake. The consensus that doctors may take risks in order to save the lifes of their patient's, however, can only be explained in light of a generally felt anxiousness about death and dying. As many questions remain, wisdom should not be forsaken.

The case of the donor

We live in a culture that is obsessed with the preservation of life. It is now regarded as routine, and perhaps even morally justifiable, to take certain risks if there is a chance that patients may benefit. Therefore, we should not reproach physicians for their irrational actions in the face of incurable and lethal diseases. While they should rightfully be expected to exercise more rationality than the masses, they are also more involved than most. Harming patients in an attempt to cure them can be excused under certain circumstances. But what about donors? It is a very different matter to harm others in an attempt to cure. This remains so even when the harm seems to be short-term and minor, and the donor's consent has been obtained.

Harm to donors

This summer the journal *Transfusion* published a series of articles on the position of the donor and donor safety. The editorial to this series reads as follows:

> "Donor safety is a critical issue in regard to the use of mobilized PBPCs. (....) Data presented in this issue of *Transfusion* indicate that the short-term administration of G-CSF is predictably associated with side effects that are generally similar to those encountered in patients undergoing autologous PBPC mobilization, but these side effects may be somewhat more pronounced, as pointed out by Stronck et al. Thus in terms of immediate side effects, the use of G-CSF to mobilize stem cells and their subsequent harvest by a single leukapheresis procedure appear to compare quite favourably with the immediate side effects and risks of marrow harvest. There are, however, additional factors to consider when mobilizing PBPCs from normal." [4]

After addressing some less pressing problems concerning venous access and thrombocytopenia, the editorial continues: "A theoretical but important concern is the potential for long term adverse effects of hematopoietic growth factor administration in normal donors. (....) *To date, there are insufficient data to evaluate this possible risk or to indicate that such a risk exists.*" Remarkably, the editorial acknowledges that current data are insufficient, then goes no further. No conclusion is drawn. From a moral point of view this is highly questionable. Rationally, if one cannot ascertain the risks involved and hence, cannot exclude long-term dangers, one should at least formulate an opinion about the appropriateness of jeopardizing 'normal' (i.e., 'healthy') donors. This discussion ends where it should begin.

The problem: the principle do no harm

There is no need to present ethicists' or lawyers' opinion on such matters. Everything that needs to be said, has been, by doctors. Consider Hippocrates for instance – though not in the Oath which is a document of minor importance likely bearing little relationship to him – but in the Book of Epidemics [in the Greek/English edition]. On page 164 Hippocrates establishes the moral essence of medicine as follows , " . . . explain the past, diagnose the present, foretell the future; practice these acts. As to diseases, make a habit of two things - to help, or at least to do no harm" (oophelein è mè blaptein) [5].

Hippocrates cautions against harming patients. It follows logically then that to harm others in an attempt to benefit patients is out of the question. An anticipated counter argument, in keeping with today's emphasis on autonomy and self-determination, might claim that the decision ought rightfully to be left to the donor. Some may insist that a prospective donor's informed consent should be all that is necessary for his cooperation.

Consent by the donor

The principle of informed consent is now a cornerstone of modern medical practice. Still, it aspires merely to ensure self-determination for patients. While self-determination may be an illusory notion, it does not follow that we should abandon efforts to achieve it. It is unlikely, however, that even an inkling of genuine consent can be obtained from family members of patients facing life-threatening circumstances. Archetypeally, they are identified as a "captive audience".

Recently the case of a very altruistic kidney donation by a kidney specialist was reported. While there is no question as to the autonomy of the decision here, the doctor certainly set a bad example by communicating a misleading message. As we cannot expect living people to donate their kidneys, doctors themselves should not be contributing to the practice. On the contrary, it would be both wiser and morally advisable to refrain from developing medical treatments which rely on the cooperation of donors yet fail to adequately safeguard their well being. It is, at least, a matter for debate.

Conclusion

Those involved in the treatment of blood cancers apparently accept that potential benefits to patients justify certain risks for donors. This is not, however, as obvious as some may think. On the contrary, although the efforts of oncologists to establish new and improved treatments may be praised, this does not warrant the use of all means. It is tragic that some patients cannot be treated effectively. It is immoral, however, to jeopardize the health of donors, even to a minor degree. This is especially important in the case of siblings or otherwise related donors given their limited freedom in refusing to cooperate. It can be argued that the long-term safety of donors represents a boundary that should not be transgressed. Hippocrates was right; it is the duty of doctors "to help, but not to harm".

References

1. Smith R. Where is the wisdom? The poverty of medical evidence. Brit Med J 1991;303: 798-99.
2. White KL. Foreword to Payer L. Medicine and culture. Varieties of treatment in the United states, England, West Germany, and France. New York. Henry Holt and Company 1988.
3. Payer L. Medicine and culture. Varieties of treatment in the United states, England, West Germany, and France. New York. Henry Holt and Company, 1988.
4. Lane ThA, Allogeneic marrow reconstitution using peripheral blood stem cells: The dawn of a new era. (Editorial). Transfusion 1996:36, 585-89 .
5. Jones WHS. Hippocrates. Vol 1. London: William Heinemann 1972:164-65.

FUTURE POTENTIAL OF CYTOKINES AND GROWTH FACTORS IN TRANSFUSION MEDICINE: WHAT NEW HORIZONS ARE THERE TO COME?

B. Löwenberg

We have come to the end of the Symposium that has highlighted various aspects of cytokines in the context of transfusion medicine, and in a broader sense the support and treatment of patients with malignant and infectious diseases. At the end we briefly flash back and focus on a disease that may serve as a model for discussing clinically relevant issues of cytokine and stem cell research. Acute myeloid leukemia is a disease where the transformed haematopoietic stem cells are unable to generate and deliver functionally differentiated cells in sufficient numbers and where the treatment has become extraordinarily intensive. The high dose intensity is applied with the objective to eradicate the ultimate residual leukemic cells and attain cure. The use of haematopoietic growth factors in adjunct to intensive chemotherapy in an effort to promote haematopoietic recovery and reduce morbidity as well as mortality and the use of haematopoietic stem cell grafts are approaches that are all being pursued in the context of the treatment of acute myeloid leukemia.

What will be the next phase?

Perhaps the new cytokines that have appeared at the firmament and that provide some promise as to the potential use for accelerating platelet regeneration may provide another possibility of better supportive care. We have learned that haematopoiesis is controlled by a number of specific regulators that act in close interaction and that permit the effective development of blood cells from immature progenitors. This process of the progressive transition of cells along successive phases of development may be mimicked in treatment. Thus, the use of defined cocktails of cytokines that drive immature cells to mature, may confer a greater therapeutic efficacy. While the first generation trials have been based on the utility of single biosynthetic regulators, the future may rather be founded upon the therapeutic use of combinations of recombinant cytokines.

Peripheral blood stem cell transplantation, as a more attractive alternative to bone marrow transplantation, is currently gaining a rapidly increasing application in clinical practice. However, it still suffers from limitations of unpredictable quality and timing of collection. For instance, one may hope that in the future it will be possible to mobilize the most primitive haematopoietic progenitors more effectively. Such advance could have a significant impact not only on autologous stem cell grafting, but also on allogeneic transplantation with simpler or better mobilization regimes. Yet another advantage of the ability to stimulate primitive haematopoietic cells with selected cocktails of cytokines relates to the possibility of expanding those cells *in vitro* and produce more “powerful” grafts. Such possibilities might also create opportunities for haematopoietic stem cell directed gene therapy for a diverse scala of haematopoietic diseases in which the molecular defect has been identified. Or for harnassing the marrow and its progeny with drug resistance genes to enhance the haematopoietic tolerance of patients with cancer and protect them against cytotoxic therapy.

Last but not least, one may foresee that the deliberate use of cytokines might help to promote haematopoietic recovery to avoid bone marrow suppression in conditions of dose escalated chemotherapy. This may for instance be of benefit to patients with leukemia who show improved survival following high-dose chemotherapy, but for the time being still at the expense of mortality, considerable morbidity and prolonged hospitalization.

DISCUSSION

B. Löwenberg and C.Th. Smit Sibinga – moderators

N.M. Heddle (Hamilton, C): Dr. Goodnough, I was wondering if you could just comment on the generalisability of the strategy of using EPO and ANH. Are there any studies you think that need to be done in other patient populations.

L.T. Goodnough (St. Louis, MO, USA): Yes, the advantage to radical prostatectomy, which I did not mention, is that there is an hour before substantial blood loss begins an initial retroperitoneal lymphnode dissection. The submission of nodes to the surgical pathologist to make sure that the cancer is local, allows us an hour to do this after induction of anaesthesia. It takes about 15 to 30 minutes for every unit of blood taken preferably along with hydroxyethyl starch or lactated Ringer's volume replacement. So it takes some time to do this. If you want to keep it inexpensive you cannot prolong operating room time otherwise it becomes very expensive. So, for joint replacement surgery we are learning how to do this, because once you induce the anaesthesia and you start orthopaedic surgery the blood loss starts much sooner than that. We have done a study in joint replacement surgery where we are doing a combination of one or two units of blood in the staging day before they go into the operating room. Before the induction of anaesthesia we are taking off two units of blood with hydroxyethyl starch replacement. After they go into the operating room and anaesthesia is induced, then very quickly after that, usually through a central line, the anaesthesiologist will take off an additional third or fourth unit. We have not analysed our data yet, but we hope that we have not prolonged operating room time. So, I think this does need to be looked at separately in other procedures, because they are a little bit different in terms of the strategy on how you might want to do this.

B. Löwenberg (Rotterdam, NL): About the scheduling of the erytropoietin treatment. Are there schedules that need to be explored to find the minimal concentration with maximal effectivity. What is known at the present time and what is your opinion about that.

L.T. Goodnough: Well I think we do need more data. The problem with the 300 units per kg daily for 14 days is it worked for regulatory approval purposes, but it is a lot of drug with a very high cost. The 4200 units per kg I estimate probably will cost about 2000 or 2500 dollars, that is too high. So, even though the labelling will read that, because that is the way the trial was done I think we badly need alternative strategies and there are investigators who are doing that. I am aware of a manuscript that has been submitted where 100 units per kg daily was given and so I think we badly need the data to show that you stimulate erythropoiesis and that you also can make it work clinically to reduce allogeneic exposure. Using smaller doses would be just fine. Our purpose in the radical prostatectomy trial is to prove the point that you can still achieve your goal with what you would call "bloodless surgery", but to do it with pharmacological doses that are cost effective.

B. Löwenberg: Is there any experience with pulses of erythropoietin with greater intervals?

L.T. Goodnough: Yes, Mark Goldberg's study[1] that I showed you. I think there is also data from Europe that is similar to this. So the concept of once a week with a higher dose has a great deal of appeal. The other advantage that European investigators have, is that they have commonly been substituting accompanying this with intravenous iron, which I did not have time to show you Francesco Mercuriali[2] and some investigators from Germany have data to show that when you give intravenous iron you facilitate the effect of erythropoietin. We do not have access to an acceptable preparation in the United States where I would recommend that.

B. Löwenberg: Do you also supply folic acid?

L.T. Goodnough: Only iron. That is actually a pretty good idea. We assume that the patient has a balanced diet and is not fully deficient, but I think folic acid supplementation is probably a good idea.

C.F. Högman (Uppsala, S): Dr. Goodnough, you indicated that you give the drug subcutaneously. I remember that it was quite often given intravenously. I wonder if you might comment on the effectivity, because I understand that giving the drug subcutaneously actually increases the effectiveness.

L.T. Goodnough: Yes, you are correct, the initial clinical trials that I showed on autologous blood donation, we gave it intravenously because we had venous access already and we felt that it would be more acceptable to patients that we did not have to give them a separate injection. But we know that the pharmacokinetics from some huge administration is superior because you have more prolonged absorption and a longer half disappearance time as it is more slowly absorbed; it circulates and it is more effective. The renal literature would suggest in trials of subcutaneous

---

1. Goldberg MA, McCutchen JW, Jove M et al. A safety and efficacy comparison study of two dosing regimens of erythropoietin alpha in patients undergoing major orthopedic surgery. Amer J Ortho 1996;258:544-52.
2. Mercuriali F, Zanella A, Barosi G et al. Use of erythropoietin to increase the volume of autologous blood donated by orthopaedic patients. Transfusion 1993; 33:55-59.

EPO compared to intravenous that you enhance the effect of erythropoietin by about 30%. So that is why now we are down to two injections preoperatively, we are giving those subcutaneously for that reason.

H. Boralessa (Brentwood, UK): Your procedure of acute isovolaemic anaemic haemodilution was it associated with any morbidity like cardiac arhythmia's or ischaemia.

L.T. Goodnough: No, we have looked at that. We ultramonitored these patients for vital signs including blood pressure and pulse. We also looked at CDP, because we have CDP lines in. You do get a mild reduction in systolic blood pressure but it is not significant. There is no associated tachycardia, there is no evidence of ischaemic episodes on ultramonitoring. So we have convinced ourselves that at least with that can be done safely and again Messmer[1] and other investigators have been using this technique for over 25 years and so we feel comfortable that it is a safe thing to do.

D.C. Dale, Seattle (WA, USA): Dr. Dupuis, I enjoyed your presentation. I wondered if you could speak a little more about what we should do or how to avoid the ethical and moral dilemmas as we try to find better ways to treat patients.

H.M. Dupuis (Leiden, NL): I would be rich if I would know that. Well I think from the point of view of morality the first thing that strikes you if you look at medicine from outside, is the absolute eagerness to do something. I mean, why would it be wrong to be a little bit more reluctant to wait and see. I know the answer of course, because you see the patient die and you want to help. It is perfectly understandable and yet I do not always understand it, for instance in the case I started with; why did they purport that there was a good reason for stimulating the brother? They must have known that the patient was almost dead and why, why, why. Why did not they just let the patient die. So, I have no recipe and I have no advice. I think a more relativating attitude towards medical practices would be the clue.

D.C. Dale: Well, I might just comment about the situation you describe. I do not know and perhaps you, too, do not know exactly what was going on there, but let us suppose that that was a patient with leukaemia, with a serious fungal infection, complicating the treatment. Let us suppose that the reason the stimulus was being given to the brother was to collect white blood cells for transfusion. Let us also suppose you knew what I know, that that might increase tenfold the chance of this person living who otherwise was almost certain to die. And let us suppose that you knew that the risk to the brother, although not known precisely, was very, very small. So, if we could improve the chance for the patient's survival tenfold and the

1. Messmer K, Kreimeier M, Intagliett A. Present state of intentional hemodilution. Eur Surg Res 1986;18:254-63.

risks to the donor were very small, either the person or the family or other people might say "go ahead". If you knew that much, would you think of this differently?

H.M. Dupuis: It is difficult, but I think it is a jump to quite an other sort of medicine, if we are going to use healthy persons in order to treat others. I mean also in the example of kidney donation we are almost sure that most people can live very long on one kidney. Yet, I think it is what in logic is a 'metabasis eis allogenos', a transition to an other sort of thinking or acting and that is what I am so worried about. So, if you pose a question so precisely as you did I would hesitate, that is true. I will agree, but nevertheless I think we must be more careful than some people are.

B. Löwenberg (Rotterdam, NL): Along the same line, this really is a dilemma that is very difficult to resolve in clinical practice. The kidney issue is perhaps a bit different. But if at some point there would be an alternative option to collect haematopoietic cells with a therapeutic advantage from a normal donor and the risks of that option for the donor would be minimal or absent, you would never be able to tell in advance. How then to resolve this dilemma. Would you say just never do it. Or is there a possibility to sort out whether this is going to be an important treatment with no risks.

H.M. Dupuis: For instance bone marrow transplantation from a donor seems to have a risk of 1 in 100,000; it is only the anaesthesia risk; then I would say yes, you should be allowed to do it. I would not think that is a real problem. But, on the other hand, every trial in this area is a bit of an endeavour without certain benefits. If I would be a doctor, I would really hesitate to involve another person in the treatment of a patient. We can exchange all sorts of parts of the body, but how far will we go? I think we all want to draw a line and then my question is, should not we draw the line a little bit nearer by than perhaps we have done sofar, if we do draw lines at all.

B. Löwenberg: But where would you draw the line if you can never absolutely predict for instance in the example we are now discussing. If you would collect white blood cells following treatment with G-CSF and consider the wealth of information available today with regard to G-CSF therapy then you would say the risk for a normal donor is probably minimal. But because there is not yet any direct experience where would you draw the line?

H.M. Dupuis: I would not do that, because of the unknown risk for the donor. I am fully willing to say that of course it is a tragedy if a person dies, but should not we sometimes accept tragedies as part of life?

C.Th. Smit Sibinga (Groningen, NL): That is a very valid point. The point in active practice of every medically qualified doctor is, it is extremely difficult to accept defeat. If you are trying to cure, trying to save life without all the emotions around it. But accepting defeat is an extremely difficult decision, and that from time to time drives our practice into certain areas which come into your area of hesitation, reluctancy. Is that really justified and as you quite rightly said it is simple to criticise once things have happened. But the point of criticising is not so much in the negativity, it should be in the positive sense to try to analyse and learn and see what we can do better for the next occasion to come. Indeed the example you gave is on both sides a tragedy having stimulated someone without taking advantage of what actually was the purpose of the stimulation. The other tragedy was in the patient self. So, it boils down to the process of awareness of how you moral-ethically handle your acting against that past history of medicine and the individual patient with the present diagnosis. With the prospect for the future that you have something in your hands which really could lead to either cure or to support at least a respectful final part of life of any individual patient. That is where the biases are. It is always funny also, I deliberately use the word funny, when respected people like you from a different field but very much involved in our medical acting try to comment "when I were a doctor". You are extremely biased in saying so, because first of all you are not – that is not a shame, it is very good – but if you would be, you would not be in your present profession and therefore not have the background, the knowledge, the wisdom through which you comment on the medical acting. The same would be true for me, you see. That is where the bias is, but it is also stimulating for the discussion.

H.M. Dupuis: My problem is not so much that doctors do harm donors, but that they think it is quite all right; so I would perhaps agree to the first case and consent and say ok, stimulate the brother. But you should know that it is something that should not be normally done and that it is something that creates a moral problem at least. But doctors seem to behave just like everything is normal. That is what really strikes me.

C.Th. Smit Sibinga: That is very true and the real meaning therefore of the '*primum est non nocere*' is much deeper and much broader than just a simple wording. We have to reflect on that every single day.

N. Choudhury (Lucknow, Ind): My first question is to Dr. Dupuis and the second to Prof. Löwenberg. Dr. Dupuis, five years back there was a problem of kidney trading in India. In some private hospitals there was a kidney trading; so government and medical profession had to put their foot down and had to prevent this kidney selling. So they go for either cadaver transplant or by a kidney from relatives. From medical point of view if that kidney can be donated by the mother that would be the best graft. This question is only complimentary to what is already discussed. The legal questions sometimes support and justify the medical question.When a cadaver kidney is not available and it is supported by the family members to give more life to this patients, how would you justify not to take the kidney from the relative.

H.M. Dupuis: That is the wrong question I would say. I would say how can we ever justify to harm a person by taking out his kidney? The only exception I would make, is that in case of a parent: because people gave life to the child as a mother or as a father. I can imagine then that you also want to donate. But for me that would be the only and really only exception. Thinking the other way round: I would never find that acceptable, because children should not donate their kidneys to their parents. Anyway I would rule it out as a practice, we should not do it. Life is very valuable, but that is also true for the donor; so I do not know who is pushing whom in this matter. Is it really the family who is pushing the doctor to take out a kidney from a living person or is it the doctor who is pushing the family?

N. Choudhury: I think it is the voluntary approach by the family members.

H.M. Dupuis: I do not believe in voluntary approach, I am sorry.

B. Löwenberg: I think the latter remark is a fundamental one, because if you say the parents are ok, then in fact you imply that it is a matter of choice, still. You say this is acceptable for me, that is not acceptable. The issue you are raising could then also work out differently in a different society with different conditions.

H.M. Dupuis: No, I am not persisting in my view in a way that I would prefer everyone to act like I would do; certainly not, but I think there are quite good arguments for a donation by a parent of a kidney to his own child. And I think that specific argument is not present in all other situations. So, that is why I would make this only exception

F. Boulton (Southampton, UK): Dr. Dupuis, I enjoyed the talk very much. I speak as a person who in the past has treated patients with leukaemia and haemophilia. Now in the blood transfusion I am much more dealing with donor care and it is a truism that even ordinary blood donors often get treated very badly by the organisations who are supposed to be looking after them. Certainly organ donors and stem cell or marrow donors in the UK are often just taken for granted by the clinical institutions which is morally indefensible. I am just repeating points that you have made and they are obvious. Very briefly one or two points which I have observed repeating what Dr. Choudhury said. I think that the situation with the kidney donors and particularly your interesting case here where the surgeon himself donated one of his kidneys for one of his patients. That is an extraordinary situation, but I think there are differences with the ethical issues that we have being faced in this symposium about the use of growth factors for non-related donors although there are obviously points in common.

Dr. Smit Sibinga talked about the difficulty of the physician, who is trying to treat. I remember many years ago really having to face this problem of what we in the UK call throwing in the towel, knowing when to stop treatment. In particular there was a young boy with leukaemia who had a brain haemorrhage in the middle of the night, a very dramatic event. I made the decision which is one of the few correct decisions I have ever made, which was not to persist in care and at autopsy he had a tiny haemorrhage in his brain stem, but it was in a vital area. That is an example of a really difficult situation to be in and all the medical training in the world will not necessarily prepare one for that specific decision when it faces you. There are ethical and cultural differences and one of the real challenges we have to recognise in this room is that, what is right for one culture is not necessary right for another. What is right for one person is not necessarily right for another. I had an opportunity to speak to Dr. Kaushansky before the meeting started. We were talking about growing platelets. The reason there is a difference in America from Europe, for in the demand of platelets we in Europe are still somewhat better placed to produce good quality platelet concentrates from ordinary donations, whereas in the States I understand there is more pressure to give TPO to donors to boost their endogenous platelet production. That is a difference of the morals of supply and demand and in culture, because there is much more acceptance I think in the States for that sort of approach, whereas I think certainly in Britain we are rather more reluctant to go that far. My last observation really is that the real interesting aspect of the interaction between the ethical debates and the clinical caring debates is: ethical debates and standing operation procedures have two dangers in common. which is that they might fossilise further developments. We have to be able to explore and go into unknown territory whenever we are making a medical advance in the treatment. Actually leukaemia is still a rare disorder in the UK 5,000 people a year die from leukaemia, but some 200,000 people die each year of other malignancies. Nevertheless we still have to be able to explore other areas and the really difficult ethical challenges how to control how to expand into these unchartered waters while still behaving in accordance with the principle of doing no harm. Sorry, I have got absolutely no answers just some extra observations.

H.M. Dupuis: I do entirely agree; only one thing that you said I cannot understand very well. You say we **have** to go on and my question would be **why**. We all know that once we have controlled one cause of death there will appear another cause of death. So, it will be an everlasting struggle and why could not it be decided to say "let us see what we can do now and let us improve our present treatments and let us leave it at that". There are so many more things to be done in the world. Why striving so much for the preservation of some more months or years in a few persons? Are not there also socially spoken better goals for science to achieve?

F. Boulton: Very, very deep waters. We are talking about individual responsibility, social responsibility; we are talking about the inevitable differences between the doctors who treat patients and who have a drive to save individual lives and their medical colleagues who are in public health medicine and also can see the whole picture of how society is spending its money on its health care. There is no easy answer, therefore I actually do believe that we must be progressive, because what is difficult now, we know will be easier in ten years time. That is the challenge of the presence. We in this room tend to be in a very narrow speciality, but your remarks are very refreshing when taking into account our individual responsibilities to society as a whole, to try to help contain the rocketing costs of health expenditure for example.

H.M. Dupuis: I would love to continue the debate, but it is not possible I am afraid.

C.Th. Smit Sibinga: One thing is sure, life ends up in death, you know. But there are other decisions to be made as well which include the respect for life and for individuals. Even if that relates to a month or two months, which may have a certain meaning to the micro-environment of that individual in all its respect.

H.J.C. de Wit (Leeuwarden, NL): Perhaps it makes thinking easier for us, workers in health care to just make a comparison with normal life. At what stage would you prevent a mother to try to get a child out of a burning house, which is something we would all do. Perhaps the problem is that in health care and for donors and specialists we have more time to think and less direct emotional action. Second, is being a donor not comparable with for example joining the voluntary fire brigade, where you know, that you join something where you will be able to save lifes or to add to health with a certain though very small risk. There are more parallels in everyday life. If you at the other side of a busy street see a child fall into a canal that cannot swim, you will cross the street, it is your citizen's duty without calculating the risk that some car will hit you. I see parallels there with deciding to be a donor or to have a relative who has a very serious life threatening illness.

H.M. Dupuis: I have many answers but the first thing that I would say is that choosing to be a fireman is entirely a voluntary choice; there is no one who is related to you in danger so you just do it, because perhaps you like to play that role or to have an important function in society. So, I doubt whether it is the same situation. The second thing is of course that it is true that our first intuition is always to save life. It is a good intuition, it is a good moral intuition, a good psychological intuition. So, it is fine but that is not what is at stake in medicine. Of course the first thought is to save life, but then immediately the second thought should be at what costs, because you say yourself you have time for reflection. I would expect then such a reflection and my problem is that I often miss that reflection.

J.I. Drayer (Alameda, CA, USA): It think it is a very worthwhile discussion and specifically when you think about these last few days in life of a patient; what you do and what you gain and I fully appreciate the concerns that you have raised there. I was a little more troubled though by the editorial that you quoted on the cytokines and I wonder whether, if you take that strict a position as you took or as the writer of the editorial took, you would never proceed in approving any future drug in the treatment of any disease. I am purposely taking the other extreme than what you have taken just to make the point. It is always, of course, possible to say I never know whether there will be long term toxicity, whether I have treated a million normal people with this medicine there will be something happening at some point in time. If you take that point of view then every pharmaceutical, biotechnology or gene therapy company would be out of business very quickly, which would also save a lot of money because we do not need the regulatory authorities and by that time maybe also need not too many doctors anymore. But is that not a little bit too extreme? Is it not that progress should be accepted against maybe the smallest risk that we all recognise and that we have to take that little bit of risk for the benefit of an improvement to a significant population that is not in the terminal stage of disease.

H.M. Dupuis: I certainly agree, I think the point of Richard Smith, the editor of the British Medical Journal[1] was that the inclination is all right and that of course we should try to work things out as well as we can, but that while doing this so many mistakes and so many errors are made. That was really his point and following that he said yes, we know so little and we do so much; that is exactly the point I wanted to make. So, I would not say we should do nothing, because I am fully aware of the benefits of medicine, but you know better than I that the real benefits of medicine can be found in for instance vaccination, in the basic care which costs 5% of all the budget and helps 95% of the people to have a longer life. So, it has something to do with focusing on the right matters and I am not sure that if you are working so specifically on such rather limited diseases, that you are on the right way at all.

J.I. Drayer: So, you would not treat any patient with an orphan disease, because this is not worthwhile; that would get you into quite a significant debate.

H.M. Dupuis: Socially spoken it is impossible, because society pushes doctors. I am sure that doctors are part of the society and that society wants doctors to do as much as possible. But I think also that doctors should take a more rational point of view and should be little more inclined to say no at some times.

N. Choudhury: With respect to the development in cytokines and growth factors how far away are we from zero risk transfusion. Is it possible in the near future, zero risk transfusion?

B. Löwenberg: Zero risk transfusion; it is a question to a prophet I think. It is difficult to make these predictions. As far as red cells are concerned, we are already a long way to achieve this goal. As far as platelets are concerned I think we will soon know, because of the availability of thrombopoietin. And as far as granulocytes are concerned that is certainly a subject that is going to be explored in the next few years as an alternative to treat patients with severe infections. We also have to see whether those transfusions will add to the arsenal of transfusions. So, we have to wait and see.

---

1. Smith R. Where is the wisdom? The poverty of medical evidence! Brit Med J 1991; 303:798-99.

C.Th. Smit Sibinga: A step forward, as we just discussed briefly, from the evident development of going into an allogeneic peripheral blood stem cell procedure, is in using cord stem cells, where you avoid the problems, where we deal with a material which is normally wasted, but which may bring a lot of other ethical questions. But there you will certainly not have a particular harm to any particular donor, while these cells as we all know do have a tremendous potential. Much more needs to be done to really become convinced of their good benefits, but maybe you could comment on that.

B. Löwenberg: Well, as far as the medical points are concerned I am happy to comment; as far as the ethical points are concerned perhaps Dr. Dupuis can comment on that. I think it is premature to make a statement on the future position of umbilical blood stem cell transplants. I would like to remind you, that we do not know yet whether these grafts are adequate to support an adult recipient. Thus, as an alternative to peripheral blood stem cell transplants, we still miss an important answer. But, there is another difference that is at least as important when we go to allogeneic peripheral blood stem cell transplants, we can use HLA fully matched grafts. Umbilical grafts are not fully matched and this introduces another potential problem. This is a question that has to be dealt with. So, it is too early to conclude on how these different modalities of transplantation actually compare. Both ways need to be pursued in parallel and in a few years we should know.

H.M. Dupuis: I see no valid argument against the use of umbilical blood I must say, because it will be thrown away anyway. So that would be a very good idea in fact.

C.Th. Smit Sibinga: Thank you very much. I think these last remarks really conclude this symposium.

INDEX

DEVELOPMENTS IN HEMATOLOGY AND IMMUNOLOGY

1. H.R. Lijnen, D. Collen and M. Verstraete (eds.): *Synthetic Substrates in Clinical Blood Coagulation Assays*. 1980 ISBN 90-247-2409-0
2. C.Th. Smit Sibinga, P.C. Das and J.O. Forfar (eds.): *Paediatrics and Blood Transfusion*. Proceedings of the 5th Annual Symposium on Blood Transfusion, organized by the Red Cross Bloodbank Groningen-Drenthe, The Netherlands (1980). 1982 ISBN 90-247-2619-0
3. N. Fabris (ed.): *Immunology and Ageing*. 1982 ISBN 90-247-2640-9
4. G. Hornstra: *Dietary Fats, Prostanoids and Arterial Thrombosis*. With an Introductory Chapter by A. Bleakley Chandler. 1982 ISBN 90-247-2667-0
5. C.Th. Smit Sibinga, P.C. Das and J.J. van Loghem (eds.): *Blood Transfusion and Problems of Bleeding*. Proceedings of the 6th Annual Symposium on Blood Transfusion, organized by the Red Cross Bloodbank Groningen-Drenthe (1981). 1982 ISBN 90-247-3058-9
6. J. Dormandy (ed.): *Red Cell Deformability and Filterability*. 1983 ISBN 0-89838-578-4
7. C.Th. Smit Sibinga, P.C. Das and H.F. Taswell (eds.): *Quality Assurance in Blood Banking and Its Clinical Impact*. Proceedings of the 7th Annual Symposium on Blood Transfusion, organized by the Red Cross Bloodbank Groningen-Drenthe (1982). 1984 ISBN 0-89838-618-7
8. A.M.H.P. van den Besselaar, H.R. Gralnick and S.M. Lewis (eds.): *Thromboplastin Calibration and Oral Anticoagulant Control*. 1984 ISBN 0-89838-637-3
9. P. Fondu and O. Thijs (eds.): *Haemostatic Failure in Liver Disease*. 1984 ISBN 0-89838-640-3
10. C.Th. Smit Sibinga, P.C. Das and G. Opelz (eds.): *Transplantation and Blood Transfusion*. Proceedings of the 8th Annual Symposium on Blood Transfusion, organized by the Red Cross Bloodbank Groningen-Drenthe (1983). 1984 ISBN 0-89838-686-1
11. H. Schmid-Schönbein, L.J. Wurzinger and R.E. Zimmerman (eds.): *Enzyme Activation in Blood-perfused Artificial Organs*. 1985 ISBN 0-89838-704-3
12. J. Dormandy (ed.): *Blood Filtration and Blood Cell Deformability*. 1985 ISBN 0-89838-714-0
13. C.Th. Smit Sibinga, P.C. Das and E. Seidl (eds.): *Plasma Fractionation and Blood Transfusion*. Proceedings of the 9th Annual Symposium on Blood Transfusion, organized by the Red Cross Bloodbank Groningen-Drenthe (1984). 1985 ISBN 0-89838-761-2
14. S. Dawids and A. Bantjes (eds.): *Blood Compatible Materials and their Testing*. 1986 ISBN 0-89838-813-9
15. C.Th. Smit Sibinga, P.C. Das and T.J. Greenwalt (eds.): *Future Developments in Blood Banking*. Proceedings of the 10th Annual Symposium on Blood Transfusion, organized by the Red Cross Bloodbank Groningen-Drenthe (1985). 1986 ISBN 0-89838-824-4
16. A. Berlin, J. Dean, M.H. Draper, E.M.B. Smith and F. Spreafico (eds.): *Immunotoxicology*. Proceedings of the International Seminar on the Immunological System as a Target for Toxic Damage – Present Status, Open Problems and Future Perspectives, in collaboration with the UNEP-ILO-WHO IPCS and the Commission of the European Communities. 1987 ISBN 0-89838-843-0

DEVELOPMENTS IN HEMATOLOGY AND IMMUNOLOGY

17. T. Ottenhoff and R. de Vries: *Recognition of M. leprae Antigens*. 1987
ISBN 0-89838-887-2
18. J.-L. Touraine, R.P. Gale and V. Kochupillai (eds.): *Fetal Liver Transplantation*. 1987
ISBN 0-89838-975-5
19. C.Th. Smit Sibinga P.C. Das and C.P. Engelfriet (eds.): *White Cells and Platelets in Blood Transfusion*. Proceedings of the 11th Annual Symposium on Blood Transfusion, organized by the Red Cross Bloodbank Groningen-Drenthe (1986). 1987
ISBN 0-89838-976-3
20. C.F.M. Hendriksen: *Laboratory Animals in Vaccine Production and Control*. 1988
ISBN 0-89838-398-6
21. C.Th. Smit Sibinga, P.C. Das and L.R. Overby (eds.): *Biotechnology in Blood Transfusion*. Proceedings of the 12th Annual Symposium on Blood Transfusion, organized by the Red Cross Bloodbank Groningen-Drenthe (1987). 1988
ISBN 0-89838-404-4
22. C.Th. Smit Sibinga, P.C. Das and C.F. Högman (eds.): *Automation in Blood Transfusion*. Proceedings of the 13th Annual Symposium on Blood Transfusion, organized by the Red Cross Bloodbank Groningen-Drenthe (1988). 1989
ISBN 0-7923-0488-8
23. S. Dawids (ed.): *Polymers: Their Properties and Blood Compatibility*. 1989
ISBN 0-7923-0491-8
24. C.Th. Smit Sibinga, P.C. Das and H.T. Meryman (eds.): *Cryopreservation and Low Temperature Biology in Blood Transfusion*. Proceedings of the 14th Annual Symposium on Blood Transfusion, organized by the Red Cross Bloodbank Groningen-Drenthe (1989). 1990 ISBN 0-7923-0908-1
25. C.Th. Smit Sibinga and L. Kater (eds.): *Advances in Haemapheresis*. Proceedings of the 3rd International Congress of the World Apheresis Association (Amsterdam, The Netherlands, 1990). 1991 ISBN 0-7923-1312-7
26. C.Th. Smit Sibinga, P.C. Das and P.M. Mannucci (eds.): *Coagulation and Blood Transfusion*. Proceedings of the 15th Annual Symposium on Blood Transfusion, organized by the Red Cross Bloodbank Groningen-Drenthe (1990). 1991
ISBN 0-7923-1331-3
27. C.Th. Smit Sibinga, P.C. Das and J.D. Cash (eds.): *Transfusion Medicine: Fact and Fiction*. Proceedings of the 16th International Symposium on Blood Transfusion, organized by the Red Cross Bloodbank Groningen-Drenthe (1991). 1992
ISBN 0-7923-1732-7
28. C.Th. Smit Sibinga, P.C. Das and T.H. The (eds.): *Immunology and Blood Transfusion*. Proceedings of the 17th International Symposium on Blood Transfusion, organized by the Red Cross Bloodbank Groningen-Drenthe (1992). 1993
ISBN 0-7923-2380-7
29. C.Th. Smit Sibinga, P.C. Das and H.J. Heiniger (eds.): *Good Manufacturing Practice in Transfusion Medicine*. Proceedings of the 18th International Symposium on Blood Transfusion, organized by the Red Cross Blood Bank Groningen-Drenthe (1993). 1994 ISBN 0-7923-3009-9

DEVELOPMENTS IN HEMATOLOGY AND IMMUNOLOGY

30. C.Th. Smit Sibinga, P.C. Das and E. Briët (eds.): *Hereditary Diseases and Blood Transfusion.* Proceedings of the 19th International Symposium on Blood Transfusion, organized by the Red Cross Blood Bank Groningen-Drenthe (1994). 1995 ISBN 0-7923-3694-1
31. C.Th. Smit Sibinga, P.C. Das and E.L. Snyder (eds.): *Trigger Factors in Transfusion Medicine.* Proceedings of the 20th International Symposium on Blood Transfusion, organized by the Red Cross Blood Bank Noord-Nederland (1995). 1996 ISBN 0-7923-4225-0
32. C.Th. Smit Sibinga, P.C. Das and B. Löwenberg (eds.): *Cytokines and Growth Factors in Blood Transfusion.* Proceedings of the 21th International Symposium on Blood Transfusion, organized by the Red Cross Blood Bank Noord-Nederland (1996). 1997 ISBN 0-7923-4787-0

KLUWER ACADEMIC PUBLISHERS – DORDRECHT / BOSTON / LONDON

GPSR Compliance

The European Union's (EU) General Product Safety Regulation (GPSR) is a set of rules that requires consumer products to be safe and our obligations to ensure this.

If you have any concerns about our products, you can contact us on ProductSafety@springernature.com

In case Publisher is established outside the EU, the EU authorized representative is:

Springer Nature Customer Service Center GmbH
Europaplatz 3
69115 Heidelberg, Germany

Batch number: 10755292

Printed by Printforce, the Netherlands